D0735906

Pocket Guide to
Prostate Cancer
Second Edition

Jeanne Held-Warmkessel
MSN, RN, AOCN®, APRN, BC

Fox Chase Cancer Center
Philadelphia, Pennsylvania

JONES AND BARTLETT PUBLISHERS
Sudbury, Massachusetts
BOSTON   TORONTO   LONDON   SINGAPORE

World Headquarters
Jones and Bartlett Publishers
40 Tall Pine Drive
Sudbury, MA 01776
978-443-5000
info@jbpub.com
www.jbpub.com

Jones and Bartlett Publishers Canada
6339 Ormindale Way
Mississauga, Ontario L5V 1J2
CANADA

Jones and Bartlett Publishers International
Barb House, Barb Mews
London W6 7PA
UK

Jones and Bartlett's books and products are available through most bookstores
and online booksellers. To contact Jones and Bartlett Publishers directly, call
800-832-0034, fax 978-443-8000, or visit our website, www.jbpub.com.

Substantial discounts on bulk quantities of Jones and Bartlett's publications are
available to corporations, professional associations, and other qualified organi-
zations. For details and specific discount information, contact the special sales
department at Jones and Bartlett via the above contact information or send an
email to specialsales@jbpub.com.

Production Credits
Executive Publisher: Christopher Davis
Associate Editor: Kathy Richardson
Production Director: Amy Rose
Production Editor: Tracey Chapman
Associate Marketing Manager: Laura Kavigian
Manufacturing and Inventory Coordinator: Amy Bacus
Composition: Graphic World
Cover Design: Kristin E. Ohlin
Printing and Binding: Kase Printing
Cover Printing: Kase Printing

6048

SEP   2007

ISBN-10: 0-7637-4046-2
ISBN-13: 978-0-7637-4046-7

Printed in the United States of America
10 09 08 07 06   10 9 8 7 6 5 4 3 2 1

Contents

Preface

Why prepare a pocket guide to prostate cancer? Clinical nurses caring for patients with prostate cancer at the bedside in the hospital, outpatient clinic, or home require an easy-to-use and up-to-date reference to assist them in direct patient care. This is the purpose of the *Pocket Guide to Prostate Cancer*. The majority of information has been abstracted from *Contemporary Issues in Prostate Cancer: A Nursing Perspective* (2nd edition) and provides the basis for the *Pocket Guide*. The reader is referred to this volume for the full text information and complete references. Research and knowledge of the nature of prostate cancer is in constant evolution. Every effort has been made to provide current information. However, the reader is reminded that new information could make the *Pocket Guide* content obsolete. Additionally, practice guidelines may vary in different institutions, regions of the country, or various practice settings.

It is my goal to provide nurses with practical information that is useful in the day-to-day care of men with prostate cancer. The content of this *Pocket Guide* is divided into four parts: Epidemiology and Screening, Disease Assessment, Treatment, and Quality of Life, in addition to an appendix that has been updated to provide access to current prostate cancer Internet resources.

This reference book would not have been possible without the foresight of Jones and Bartlett Publishers in requesting this *Pocket Guide*. I would like to thank Kathy Richardson for her support throughout manuscript development. In addition I would like to acknowledge those who assisted in the development of this publication—Kate Hennessy and Mark Goodin. The content provided by the chapter authors of *Contemporary Issues in Prostate Cancer: A Nursing Perspective* (2nd edition) was invaluable. I therefore wish to acknowledge the following nurses and physicians for their expertise in the areas of prostate cancer nursing and patient care:

Denise Bickert, MSN, RN, CNOR
Carol Blecher, MS, RN, AOCN
Maria DeVito Brouch, MS, RN, AOCN
Jennifer Cash, MS, ARPN
Elissa C. Clayton, MS, ARPN
Mary Collins, MSN, RN, OCN

Georgia M. Decker, MS, RN, CS-ANP, CN, AOCN
Cynthia R. King, PhD, NP, MSN, RN, CS, FAAN
Alberto Mizrachi, MD
Maureen E. O'Rourke, PhD, RN
Susan K. Roethke, MSN, CRNP, AOCN
Laura Stempkowski, MS, CUNP, AOCN
William Tester, MD, FACP
Heidi M. Volpe, MSN, RN, CCRA
Anne Robin Waldman, MSN, RN, C, AOCN
Scott V. Watkins, MD

Support and understanding by family, friends, and coworkers was essential during the content preparation. I thank my husband, Brian Warmkessel, my mother, Irene Held, and my parrot, Mango, for understanding the amount of time needed to prepare text content. I also wish to acknowledge the Department of Nursing at Fox Chase Cancer Center, including Joanne M. Hambleton, MSN, RN, CNA, and Anne Jadwin, MSN, RN, AOCN.

Part I

Epidemiology and Screening

Epidemiology, Risk Factors, and Prevention Strategies

EPIDEMIOLOGY AND ETIOLOGY
Introduction[1-12]

Incidence rates
- Estimated new cancer cases in 2005: 232,090
- Estimated cancer deaths in 2005: 30,350
- Declined between 1992 and 1995 with an increased rate of diagnosis from 1995 to 2001. Aging population is expected to increase incidence of disease.
- Increased rate of diagnosis may also be due to transurethral resections, increased routine prostate biopsies, and increased number of biopsy specimens obtained from each patient.

Mortality rates
- Declining at a rate of 4.1% each year from 1994 to 2001
  - Rate for white men is 4.2%
  - Rate for African-American men is 2.7%
- 32 deaths per 100,000 men
- Rates are highest for American Indians/Native Americans, African-American, Hispanic white men.
- Disparity may be related to low socioeconomic status, lack of health insurance, low literacy rates, and lack of access to health care.
- May be declining due to use of PSA screening and testing

Molecular Genetics[13-56]
- Wide range of behavior from indolent to aggressive, androgen dependent to androgen independent
- Rare germ line inheritable mutations
- More common are somatic noninheritable cell mutations (see **Table 1–1**)
- Androgen receptor (AR) mutations changes in the CAG repeats in the AR gene could predispose men of different races to an increased risk (shortened CAG repeats) or a lower risk (longer CAG repeats). More research is needed to determine the prostate cancer risk related to short CAG repeats.
- CYP17 gene on chromosome 10q24.3 encodes for an enzyme that participates in the synthesis of androgens; polymorphism is probably not a major prostate cancer risk factor.
- SRD5A2 gene encodes for type II 5α-reductase; undetermined if polymorphism is a prostate cancer risk factor because of conflicting research study results
- PTEN tumor-suppressor gene on chromosome 10q23 encodes for a phosphatase; mutations are frequently found in human cancers and may be associated with prostate cancer progression. This gene may reduce p27 levels resulting in increased prostate cancer cell growth and decreased prostate cancer apoptosis.

- NKX3.1 gene located on chromosome 8p21 has an essential role in prostate cell differentiation and cell growth; may be a "gatekeeper" gene. Gene loss occurs early in the carcinogenic process (63% of PIN lesions, 90% of prostate cancer lesions).[42–43]
- CDKN1B gene on 12p11–13 is a member of Cip/Kip family and plays a role in cell cycle and G-1 phase arrest. Encodes a cycline-dependent kinase inhibitor called p27. Reduced p27 levels are seen in prostate cancer with a poor prognosis. Has been found in some studies of hereditary prostate cancer families.
- GSTP1 may be a "caretaker" gene that repairs DNA. Absent in PIN and prostate cancer cells.
- Multiple genes and environmental factors are probably involved in prostate cancer carcinogenesis.

Precursor Lesions[15, 57–66]

Prostatic intraepithelial neoplasia (PIN)
- Two types identified—low-grade PIN (LGPIN) and high-grade PIN (HGPIN)
- LGPIN is not believed to increase prostate cancer risk.
- HGPIN is associated with prostate cancer and is a premalignant lesion. It is often associated with prostate cancer and adjacent to it in prostate specimens. Other precursor lesions await discovery.
- Presence of HGPIN indicates the need for repeated biopsies.

Atypical small acinar proliferation (ASAP) or atypical adenomatous hyperplasia (AAH)
- May not be a premalignant lesion
- If present with or adjacent to HGPIN, risk of prostate cancer on repeat biopsy is higher than with HGPIN alone.

Proliferative inflammatory atrophy (PIA)
- May be a precursor to PIN and prostate cancer
- Associated with inflammation
- Occurs in gland periphery
- Often alongside HGPIN, prostate cancer, or both
- More research is needed on association between PIA, PIN, and prostate cancer.

TABLE 1–1 Selected Somatic Gene Alterations Implicated in Prostate Carcinogenesis

Gene	Chromosome Location	Proposed Function
AR	Xq11-12	Binding of androgens and translocation to nucleus for DNA binding; transactivation of gene with androgen responsive elements
CYP17	10q24.3	Testicular synthesis of androgens
SRD5A2	2p23	Catalyzes the irreversible conversion of testosterone to DHT
PTEN	10q23	Inhibits p13/Akt cell-surviving signals
NKX3.1	8p21	Regulates cell growth
GSTP1	11q13	Carcinogen detoxifications
CDKN1B	12p13	Cell cycle control

Source: Clayton EC. Epidemiology, risk factors, and prevention strategies. In Held-Warmkessel, J. ed. *Contemporary issues in prostate cancer: A Nursing Perspective* (2nd ed). Jones and Barlett Publishers, 2006, 1–43.

RISK FACTORS
(See **Table 1–2.**)

Age

- Disease of older men

Racial and Ethnic Factors[9, 67–76]

- Incidence varies widely among different groups
- Latent prostate cancer rates in different countries vary little

African-American men have
- Higher incidence rate of PIN
- Higher PSA levels
- Higher Gleason scores
- Higher prostate cancer incidence rate
- Higher mortality rate
- Diagnosis at later stage
- Potentially more aggressive disease
- Worse prognosis and poorer survival
- Higher testosterone levels, which may play a role in the increased incidence rate

TABLE 1–2 Risk Factors

Risk Factor	Epidemiologic Evidence	Reference
Age	Strong	11
Race and ethnicity	Strong	11
Family history	Strong	15, 133, 135
Tobacco	Overall weak	196
	Stronger evidence for association with aggressive disease	197–201
Alcohol	Weak	202–204
Occupation exposure	Inconsistent	
Organochlorine pesticides		219–220
Endogenous hormonal steroids	Weak	222–228, 231, 244–248
Sexuality issues	Inconsistent	251–256
Obesity	Inconsistent	263–269
Physical activity	Inconsistent	271, 281–283
Dietary fat	Inconsistent	289–291
Vitamin E	Strong—phase 3 clinical trials ongoing	303, 304, 306
Vitamin A	Weak	308
Lycopene	Preliminary—phase 1 trial ongoing	312–317
Selenium	Strong—phase 3 clinical trial ongoing	319–325
Isoflavones	Preliminary—phase 2 trial ongoing	315, 336–338
Tea polyphenols	Preliminary	343–345

Source: Clayton EC. Epidemiology, risk factors, and prevention strategies. In: Held-Warmkessel, J., ed. *Contemporary Issues in Prostate Cancer: A Nursing Perspective* (2nd ed). Jones and Bartlett Publishers, 2006, 1–43.

White men have
- Second highest incidence rate

Groups with lower incidence rates
- Native American
- Asian
- Emigration to the United States increases incidence in people from low risk countries.

Family History[14, 77–90]

Risk of prostate cancer increased among men with
- First-degree relative with prostate cancer diagnosis
- Increased number of first-degree family members with prostate cancer diagnosis
- Brother (higher risk) or father with prostate cancer diagnosis
- Similar findings among different ethnic groups
- Recurrence risk higher if diagnosed under age 65 years

Definition of inherited prostate cancer[83]
- Three or more males with prostate cancer in one nuclear family
- Three successive generations of patients with prostate cancer from the maternal or paternal line
- Two or more patients with prostate cancer under age 55 years

Other pertinent items in the family history
- Monozygotic twins may have a higher incidence of prostate cancer than dizygotic twins.
- Prostate cancer may have an autosomal dominance pattern or an X-linked or recessive component.
- Much more research is needed on the genetics and family risk of prostate cancer.

Inherited Genetic Susceptibility[14, 91–101]

HPC1 region and RNASE1 gene
- Located at 1q24–25
- May be a major prostate cancer susceptibility locus

8p22–23 region, MSR1 gene, and PINX1 gene
- May play a role in familial prostate cancer

HPC2 region and ELCA 2 gene
- Located at 17p11
- Could play an undetermined role in prostate cancer susceptibility

PCAP
- Located at 1q42–43, role undetermined

HPC20
- Located at 20q13, role undetermined

HPCX
- Located at Xq27–28
- Maternal transmission to male offspring
- Role undetermined

CAPB region
- Located on chromosome 1q36

Much more research is needed on identifying and determining the role and function of candidate susceptibility genes.

Smoking and Ethanol Use

- Long smoking history may increase prostate cancer risk.
- Smoking may reduce survival in diagnosed patients.
- Alcohol consumption does not appear to play a major role.

Occupational and Exposure History[109–114]

Potential risk factors
- Being employed as a farm worker
- Exposure to pesticides, including exposure to organochlorine, organophosphate, fumigants, and triazine herbicides

Hormonal and Steroid Factors[115–125]

- Normal prostate tissue is androgen dependent.
- Prostate cancer regression occurs after removal of androgens.
- Prostate cancer development is androgen dependent.
- Role of estrogen is unclear and requires more research.
- Role of insulin and leptin requires more research as does the role of vitamin D.
- More research is needed on the relationship between hormones and prostate cancer risk, disease progression, and development of androgen-independent disease.

Sexuality Issues[126–128]

- Viruses and other sexually transmitted infections (STIs)
- Risk of prostate cancer may be increased by infection with human papillomavirus types 18 or 16, syphilis, gonorrhea, and other STIs.

Body Size and Energy Expenditure

- Weight, body mass index (BMI), weight gain, physical activity, type of physical activity, energy expenditure, and body stature all require additional research in their relationship to prostate cancer, prostate cancer family history and incidence, and the affect on hormone levels and immunity function.

Dietary Factors[129–161]

- Increased risk of prostate cancer may be associated with high-fat diets, high-animal-fat diets, high-calorie diets, and red meat consumption
- Role of the following vitamins or dietary compounds:
  - Higher intake of cooked tomatoes and tomato products appears to have a role in reducing prostate cancer risk. The role of lycopene is not as strong.
  - Vitamin E supplements may decrease risk. Currently being researched in the Selenium and Vitamin E Cancer Prevention Trial (SELECT).
  - Selenium is a trace element with antioxidant activity.
    - Reduces prostate cancer risk especially in men with a PSA < 4 ng/mL and in men with low baseline selenium levels
    - Promotes G1 arrest and apoptosis
- Soy phytoestrogens (isoflavones) may have a number of affects on cell cycle, angiogenesis, pathway signaling, and enzyme activity.
  - May have a protective affect that reduces risk of prostate cancer
  - A high consumption of soybeans and soy products may reduce prostate cancer risk, but more research is needed.

- Green tea has antioxidant properties.
  - Promotes apoptosis and cell cycle arrest and reduces androgen activity
  - Increased green tea consumption may reduce the risk of prostate cancer, but more research is needed.

PREVENTION[162–165]

Hormonal Approaches

- The Prostate Cancer Prevention Trial—Tested the effects of blocking the enzyme 5α-reductase, which is responsible for conversion of testosterone to DHT, with finasteride 5 mg/day in a placebo-controlled clinical trial lasting 7 years. Patients treated with finasteride had a 24.8% reduction in prostate cancer incidence.[162] In those patients who did develop prostate cancer, the Gleason score was higher.
- Multiple clinical trials are underway using different agents such as dustasteride, finasteride, or toremifine.

Dietary Components[131, 140, 166–169]

- Isoflavones and genestein currently being investigated in two prospective randomized placebo-controlled clinical trials.
- Vitamin E—In the Alpha-Tocopherol, Beta-Carotene Cancer Prevention Trial, a 34% reduction in prostate cancer incidence was observed in men receiving alpha-tocopherol.
- The National Prevention of Cancer Study—Prostate cancer risk reduced by 50% in those subjects taking selenium-enriched yeast.
- Health Care Professionals Follow-up Study showed that vitamin E reduced prostate cancer risk in some subjects.
- Currently being investigated in:
- The Physician's Health Study II, a randomized double-blind, placebo-controlled trial to evaluate the effect of different vitamins (E, C, and multivitamins) on prostate cancer incidence
- SELECT trial to evaluate the effect of vitamin E and selenium, alone and in combination, on prostate cancer incidence
- Lycopene and tomato products are currently in early clinical trials.

NURSING IMPLICATIONS[170]

- Provide risk factor information.
- Identify at-risk individuals and groups needing screening.
- Perform health assessments.
- Provide education regarding risks versus benefits of screening and follow-up.
- Monitor research findings.
- Promote participation of individuals or groups in screening.
- Make referrals to genetic counselors and family risk assessment programs.
- Encourage participation in family registries.

References

1. Jemal A, Murray T, Ward E, et al. Cancer statistics, 2005. *CA Cancer J Clin.* 2005;55:10–30.
2. Jemal A, Clegg LX, Ward E. Annual report to the nation on the status of cancer, 1975–2001, with a special feature regarding survival. *Cancer.* 2004;101:3–27.
3. Walsh P. Urological oncology: prostate cancer. *J Urol.* 2004;172:392–398.

4. Potosky AL, Kessler L, Grindley G, et al. Rise in prostatic cancer incidence associated with increased use of transurethral resection. *J Natl Cancer Inst.* 1990; 82:1624–1628.
5. Merrill RM, Feuer EJ, Warren JL, et al. Role of transurethral resection of the prostate in population-based prostate cancer incidence rates. *Am J Epidemiol.* 1999;150:848–860.
6. Hodge KK, Mcneal JE, Terris MK, Stamey TA. Random systematic versus directed ultrasound-guided transrectal core-biopsies of the prostate. *J Urol.* 1989;142:71–74.
7. Presti JR, O'Dowd GJ, Miller MC, et al. Extended peripheral zone biopsy schemes increase cancer detection rates and minimize variance in prostate-specific antigen and age-related cancer rates; results of a community multi-practice study. *J Urol.* 2003;169:125–129.
8. Stewart CS, Leibovich BC, Weaver AL, Leiber MM. Prostate cancer diagnosis using a saturation biopsy technique after previous negative sextant biopsies. *J Urol.* 2001;166:86–91.
9. Ries LAG, Eisner MP, Kosary CL, et al, eds. *SEER Cancer Statistics Review, 1975–2001.* Bethesda, MD: National Cancer Institute; 2004. Available at: http://seer.cancer.gov/csr/1975_2001/. Accessed May 15, 2006.
10. Bennett CL, Ferreira MR, Davis TC, et al. Relation between literacy, race, and stage of presentation among low-income patients with prostate cancer. *J Clin Oncol.* 1998;16:3101–3104.
11. Legler J, Feuer E, Potosky A, et al. The role of prostate-specific antigen (PSA) testing patterns in the recent prostate incidence cancer decline in the USA. *Cancer Causes Control.* 1998;9:519–527.
12. Etzioni R, Berry KM, Legler JM. PSA testing in the US population: analysis of Medicare claims from 1991–1998. *Urology.* 2002;59:251–255.
13. Nussbaum RL, McInnes RR, Willard HF, eds. *Thompson & Thompson Genetics in Medicine.* 6th ed. Philadelphia, Pa: WB Saunders Company; 2001:311–333.
14. Schaid DJ. The complex epidemiology of prostate cancer. *Hum Mol Genet.* 2004;13 (special issue 1):R103–R121.
15. DeMarzo AM, Nelson G, Issacs WB, Epstein JI. Pathological and molecular aspects of prostate cancer. *Lancet.* 2003;361:955–964.
16. Nelson WG, DeMarzo AM, Isaacs WB. Prostate Cancer. *N Engl J Med.* 2003;349: 366–381.
17. Irvine RA, Ma H, Favaloro JM, et al. Inhibition of p160-mediated coactivation with increasing androgen receptor polyglutamine length. *Hum Mol Genet.* 2000; 9:267–274.
18. Beilin J, Ball EM, Favaloro JM, Zajac JD. Effect of androgen receptor CAG repeat polymorphism on transcriptional activity: specificity in prostate and non-prostate cell lines. *J Mol Endocrinol.* 2000;25:85–96.
19. Edwards A, Hammond HA, Jin L, et al. Genetic variation at five trimeric and tetrameric tandem repeat loci in four human population groups. *Genomics.* 1992;12:241–253.
20. Irvine RA, Yu MC, Ross RK, Coetzee GA. The CAG and GGC microsatellites of the androgen receptor gene are in linkage disequilibrium in men with prostate cancer. *Cancer Res.* 1995;55:1937–1940.
21. Bennett CL, Price DK, Kim S, et al. Racial variation in CAG repeat lengths within the androgen receptor gene among prostate cancer patients of lower socioeconomic status. *J Clin Oncol.* 2002;20:3599–3604.

22. Latil AG, Azzouzi R, Cancel GS, et al. Prostate carcinoma risk and allelic variants of genes involved in androgen biosynthesis and metabolism pathways. *Cancer.* 2001;92:1130–1137.
23. Hsing AW, Gao YT, Wu , et al. Polymorphic CAG and GGN repeat lengths in the androgen receptor gene and prostate cancer risk: a population-based case-control study in China. *Cancer Res.* 2000;60:5111–5116.
24. Hakimi JM, Schoenberg MP, Rondinelli R, et al. Androgen receptor variants with short glutamine or glycine repeats may identify unique sub-populations of men with prostate cancer. *Clin Cancer Res.* 1997;3:1599–1608.
25. Giovannucci E, Stampfer MJ, Krithivas, K et al. The CAG repeat within the androgen receptor gene and its relationship to prostate cancer. *Proc Natl Acad Sci USA.* 1997;94:3320–3323.
26. Stanford JL, Just JJ, Gibbs M, et al. Polymorphic repeats in the androgen receptor gene: molecular markers of prostate cancer risk. *Cancer Res.* 1997;57:1194–1198.
27. Lewis DF, Lee-Robichaud P. Molecular modeling of steroidogenic cytochromes P450 from families CYP11, CYP17, CYP19 and CYP21 based on the CYP102 crystal structure. *J Steroid Biochem Mol Biol.* 1998;66:217–233.
28. Ntais C, Polycarpou A, Ioannidis JP. Association of the CYP17 gene polymorphism with the risk of prostate cancer: a meta-analysis. *Cancer Epidemiol Biomarkers Prev.* 2003;12:120–126.
29. Makridakis NM, Ross RK, Pike MC, et al. Association of missense substitution in SRD5A2 gene with prostate cancer in African American and Hispanic men in Los Angeles, USA. *Lancet.* 1999;354:975–978.
30. Nam RK, Toi A, Vesprini D, et al. V89L polymorphism of type-2, 5-alpha reductase enzyme gene predicts prostate cancer and progression. *Urology.* 2001;57:199–204.
31. Mononen N, Ikonen T, Syrjakoski K, et al. A mis-sense substitution A49T in steroid 5-alpha-reductase gene (SRD5A2) is not associated with prostate cancer in Finland. *Br J Cancer.* 2001;10:1344–1347.
32. Lin H-K, Hu Y-C, Lee DK. Regulation of androgen receptor signaling by PTEN (phoshatase and tensin homolog deleted on chromosome 10) tumor suppressor through distinct mechanisms in prostate cancer cells. *Mol Endocrinol.* 2004;18:2409–2423.
33. Li J, Yen C, Liaw D, et al. PTEN, a putative protein tryosine phosphatase gene mutated in human brain, breast and prostate cancer. *Science.* 1997;275:1943–1947.
34. Teng DH, Hu R, Lin H, et al. MMAC1/PTEN mutations in primary tumor specimens and tumor cell lines. *Cancer Res.* 1997;57:5221–5225.
35. Myers MP, Pass I, Batty IH, et al. The lipid phosphatase activity of PTEN is critical for tumor suppression function. *Proc Natl Acad Sci USA.* 1998;95:13513–13518.
36. Suzuki H, Freije D, Nusskern DR, et al. Interfocal heterogeneity of PTEN/MMAC1 gene alterations in multiple metastatic prostate cancer tissues. *Cancer Res.* 1998;58:204–209.
37. Ramaswamy S, Nakamura N, Vazquez F, et al. Regulation of G1 progression by PTEN tumor suppression protein is linked to inhibition of the phoshatidylinositol 3-kinase/Akt pathway. *Proc Natl Acad Sci USA.* 1999;96:2110–2115.
38. Sun H, Lesche R, Li DM, et al. PTEN modulates cell cycle progression and cell survival by regulating phoshatidylinositol 3,4,5,-triphosphate and Akt/protein kinase B signaling pathway. *Proc Natl Acad Sci USA.* 1999;96:6199–6204.
39. McMenamin ME, Soung P, Perea S, et al. Loss of PTEN expression in paraffin-embedded primary prostate cancer correlates with high Gleason score and advanced stage. *Cancer Res.* 1999;59:4291–4296.

40. Bieberich CJ, Fujita K, He WW, Jay G. Prostate specific and androgen-dependent expression of a novel homeobox gene. *J Biol Chem.* 1996;271:31779–31782.
41. Sciavolino PJ, Abrams EW, Yang L, et al. Tissue-specific expression of murine Nkx.3 in the male urogenital system. *Dev Dyn.* 1997;209:127–138.
42. Emmert-Buck MR, Vocke CD, Pozzatti RO, et al. Allelic loss on chromosome 8p12–21 in microdissected prostatic intraepithelial neoplasia. *Cancer Res.* 1995; 55:2959–2962
43. He WW, Sciavolino PJ, Wing J, et al. A novel human prostate-specific, androgen-regulated homeobox gene (NKX.3.1) that maps to 8p21, a region frequently deleted in prostate cancer. *Genomics.* 1997;43:69–77.
44. Tsihlias J, Kapusta LR, DeBoer , et al. Loss of cyclin-dependent kinase inhibitor p27Kip1 is a novel prognostic factor in localized human prostate adenocarcinoma. *Cancer Res.* 1998;58:542–548.
45. Cote RJ, Shi Y, Groshen S, et al. Association of p27Kip1 levels with recurrence and survival in patients with stage C prostate carcinoma. *J Natl Cancer Inst.* 1998;90:916–920.
46. Yang RM, Naitoh J, Murphy M, et al. Low p27 expression predicts poor disease-free survival in patients with prostate cancer. *J Urol.* 1998;159:941–945.
47. Suarez BK, Lin J, Burmester JK, et al. A genome screen of muliplex sibships with prostate cancer. *Am J Hum Genet.* 2000;66:933–944.
48. Hsieh CL, Oakley-Girvan I, Balise R, et al. A genome screen of families with multiple cases of prostate cancer: evidence of genetic heterogenicity. *Am J Hum Genet.* 2001;69:148–158.
49. Chang B, Zheng S, Isaacs S, et al. A polymorphism in the CDKN1B gene is associated with increased risk of hereditary prostate cancer. *Cancer Res.* 2004;64: 1997–1999.
50. Kinzler KW, Vogelstein B. Cancer-susceptibility genes: gatekeepers and caretakers. *Nature.* 1997;386;763–761.
51. Shirai T, Sano M, Tamano S, et al. The prostate: a target for carcinogenicity of 2-amino-1-methyl-6-phenylimidazol (4,5-*b*)pyridine (PhPI) derived from cooked foods. *Cancer Res.* 1997;57:195–198.
52. Rebbeck TR. Molecular epidemiology of the human glutathione S-transferase genotypes GSTM1 and GSTT1 in cancer susceptibility. *Cancer Epidemiol Biomarkers Prev.* 1997;6:733–743.
53. Harries LW, Stubbins MJ, Forman D, et al. Identification of genetic polymorphisms at the glutathione S-transferase pi locus and association with susceptibility to bladder, testicular and prostate cancer. *Carcinogenesis.* 1997;18:641–644.
54. Lin X, Tascilar M, Lee WH, et al. GSTP1 CpG island hypermethylation is responsible for the absence of GSTP1 expression in human prostate cancer cells. *Am J Pathol.* 2001;159:1815–1826.
55. Millar DS, Ow KK, Paul CL, et al. Detailed methylation analysis of the glutathione S-transferase pi (GSTP1). *Oncogene.* 1999;18:1313–1324.
56. Brooks JD, Weinstein M, Lin X, et al. CG island methylation changes near GSTP1 gene in prostatic intraepithelial neoplasia. *Cancer Epidemiol Biomarkers Prev.* 1998;7:531–536.
57. Davidson D, Bostwick DG, Qian J, et al. Prostatic intraepithelial neoplasia is a risk factor for adenocarcinoma: predictive accuracy in needle biopsies. *J Urol.* 1995;154: 1295–1299.
58. Weinstein MH, Epstein JI. Significance of high-grade prostatic intraepithelial neoplasia (PIN) on needle biopsy. *Hum Pathol.* 1993;24:624–629.

59. Haggman MJ, Macoska JA, Wojno KJ, Oesterling JE. The relationship between prostatic intraepithelial neoplasia and prostate cancer: critical issues. *J Urol.* 1997;158:12–22.
60. Ickowski KA, MacLennan GT, Bostwick DG. Atypical small acinar proliferation suspicious for malignancy in prostate needle biopsies: clinical significance in 33 cases. *Am J Surg Pathol.* 1997;21:1489–1495.
61. Alfikafi NF, Brendler CB, Gerer GS, et al. High-grade prostatic intraepithelial neoplasia with adjacent atypia is associated with a higher incidence of cancer on subsequent needle biopsy than high-grade intraepithelial neoplasia alone. *Urology.* 2001;57:296–300.
62. Meng MV, Shinohara K, Grossfwld GD. Significance of high-grade intraepithelial neoplasia on prostate biopsy. *Urol Oncol.* 2003;21:145–151.
63. Coussens LM, Werb Z. Inflammation and cancer. *Nature.* 2002;420:860–867.
64. DeMarzo AM, Marchi VL, Epstein JI. Proliferative inflammatory atrophy of the prostate: implications for prostatic carcinogenesis. *Am J Pathol.* 1999;155:1985–1992.
65. Ruska KM, Sauvageot J, Epstein JI. Histology and cellular kinetics of prostatic atrophy. *Am J Surg Pathol.* 1998;22:1073–1077.
66. Putzi MJ, De Marzo AM. Morphologic transitions between proliferative inflammatory atrophy and high-grade prostatic intraepithelial neoplasia. *Urology.* 2000;56:828–832.
67. Breslow N, Chan CW, Dhom G, et al. Latent carcinoma of the prostate in seven areas. *Int J Cancer.* 1977;20:680–688.
68. Sakr WA, Grignon DJ, Haas GP. Epidemiology of high grade intraepithelial neoplasia. *Pathol Res Pract.* 1995;191:838–841.
69. Moul J, Sesterhenn I, Connelly R, et al. Prostate-specific antigen values at the time of prostate cancer diagnosis in African-American men. *JAMA.* 1995;274:1277–1281.
70. Powell I, Banerjee M, Sakr WA, et al. Should African-American men be tested for prostate carcinoma at an earlier age than white men? *Cancer.* 1999;85:472–477.
71. Thompson I, Tangen C, Toclher A, et al. Association of African-American ethnic background with survival in men with metastatic prostate cancer. *J Natl Cancer Inst.* 2001;93:219–225.
72. Ross R, Bernstein L, Judd H, et al. Serum testosterone levels in healthy black and white men. *J Natl Cancer Inst.* 1986;76:45–48.
73. Ross RK, Bernstein L, Lobo R, et al. 5-alpha-reductase activity and risk of prostate cancer among Japanese and US white and black males. *Lancet.* 1992;339:887–889.
74. Ellis L, Nyorg H. Racial/ethnic variations in male testosterone levels: a probable contributor to group differences in health. *Steroids.* 1992;57:72–75.
75. Whittenmore AS, Kolonel LN, Wu AH, et al. Prostate cancer in relation to diet, physical activity, and body size in blacks, whites and Asians in the United States and Canada. *J Natl Cancer Inst.* 1995;87:652–661.
76. Shimizu H, Ross RK, Bernstein L, et al. Cancers of the prostate and breast among Japanese and white immigrants in Los Angeles County. *Br J Cancer.* 1991;63:963–966.
77. Steinberg GD, Carter BS, Beaty TH, et al. Family history and the risk of prostate cancer. *Prostate.* 1990;17:337–347.
78. Johns LE, Houlston RS. A systematic review and meta-analysis of familial prostate cancer risk. *BJU Int.* 2003;91:789–794.
79. Zeegers M, Jellema A, Ostrer H. Empiric risk of prostate carcinoma for relatives of patients with prostate carcinoma: a meta-analysis. *Cancer.* 2003;97:1894–1903.

80. Whittemore AS, Wu AH, Kolonel LN, et al. Family history and prostate cancer risk in black, white, and Asian men in the United States and Canada. *Am J Epidemiol.* 1995;141:732–740.
81. Cunningham G, Ashton C, Annegers J, et al. Familial aggregation of prostate cancer in African-Americans and White Americans. *Prostate.* 2003;56:256–262.
82. Gronberg H, Damber L, Damber J, Iselius L. Support for dominant inheritance. *Am J Epidemiol.* 1997;146:552–557.
83. Carter BS, Bova GS, Beaty TH, et al. Hereditary prostate cancer: epidemiologic and clinical features. *J Urol.* 1993;150:797–802.
84. Lichtenstein P, Holm NV, Verkaslo P, et al. Environmental and heritable factors in the causation of cancer—analyses of cohorts of twins from Sweden, Denmark, and Finland. *N England J Med.* 2000;343:78–85.
85. Risch N. The genetic epidemiology of cancer: interpreting familial and twin studies and their implications for molecular genetic approaches. *Cancer Epidemiol Biomark Prev.* 2001;10:733–741.
86. Carter BS, Beaty TH, Steinberg GD, et al. Mendelian inheritance of familial prostate cancer. *Proc Natl Acad Sci USA.* 1992;89:3367–3371.
87. Schaid DJ, MacDonnell SK, Blute ML, Thibodeau SN. Evidence for autosomal dominant inheritance of prostate cancer. *Am J Hum Genet.* 1998;62:1425–1438.
88. Verbage BA, Baffoe-Bonnie AB, Baglietto L, et al. Autosomal dominant inheritance of prostate cancer: a confirmatory study. *Urology.* 2001;57:97–101.
89. Valeri A, Briollais L, Azzouzi R, et al. Segregation analysis of prostate cancer in France: evidence for autosomal dominant inheritance and residual brother-brother dependence. *Ann Hum Genet.* 2003;67:125–137.
90. Gronberg H, Damber L, Damber J, Iselius L. Support for dominant inheritance. *Am J Epidemiol* 1997;146:552–557.
91. Smith JR, Freije D, Carpeten JD, et al. Major susceptibility locus for prostate cancer on chromosome 1 suggested by genome-wide search. *Science.* 1996;274:1371–1374.
92. Xu J, Zheng SL, Hawkins GA, et al. Linkage and association studies of prostate cancer susceptibility: evidence for linkage at 8p22–23. *Am J Hum Genet.* 2001;69:341–350.
93. Wiklund F, Jonsson BA, Goransson IB. Linkage analysis of prostate cancer susceptibility: confirmation of linkage at 8p22–23. *Hum Genet.* 2003;112:414–418.
94. Tavtigian SV, Simard J, Teng DH, et al. A candidate prostate cancer susceptibility gene at chromosome 17p. *Nat Genet.* 2001;27:172–180.
95. Xu J, Zheng SL, Carpten JD, et al. Evaluation of linkage association of HPC2/ELCA2 in patients with familial or sporadic prostate cancer. *Am J Hum Genet.* 2001;68:901–911.
96. Rokman A, Ikonen T, Mononen N, et al. ELCA2/HPC2 involvement in hereditary and sporadic prostate cancer. *Cancer Res.* 2001;61:6038–6041.
97. Suarez BK, Gerhard DS, Lin J, et al. Polymorphisms in the prostate cancer susceptibility gene HPC2/ELCA2 in multiplex families and healthy controls. *Cancer Res.* 2001;61:4982–4984.
98. Shea PR, Ferrell RE, Patrick AL, et al. ELCA2 and prostate cancer risk in Afro-Caribbeans of Tobago. *Hum Genet.* 2002;111:398–400.
99. Berthon P, Valeri A, Cohen-Akenine A, et al. Predisposing gene for early onset prostate cancer, localized on chromosome 1q42.2–43. *Am J Hum Genet.* 1998;62:1416–1424.
100. Xu J, Meyers D, Freije D, et al. Evidence for a prostate susceptibility locus on the X chromosome. *Nat Genet.* 1998;20:175–179.

101. Gibbs M, Stanford JL, McIndoe RA, et al. Evidence for a rare prostate cancer-susceptibility locus at chromosome 1p36. *Am J Hum Genet.* 1999;64:776–787.
102. Hickey K, Do KA, Green A. Smoking and prostate cancer. *Epidemiol Rev.* 2001;23:115–125.
103. Plaskon LA, Penson DF, Thomas LV, Stanford JL. Cigarette smoking and risk of prostate cancer in middle-aged men. *Cancer Epidemiol Biomarkers Prev.* 2003;12:604–609.
104. Giovannucci E, Rimm EB, Asheria A, et al. Smoking and risk of total and fatal prostate cancer in United States health care professionals. *Cancer Epidemiol Biomark Prev.* 1999;8:277–282.
105. Rodriguez C, Tatham LM, Thun MJ, et al. Smoking and fatal prostate cancer in a large cohort of adult men. *Am J Epidemiol.* 1997;145:466–475.
106. Couglin SS, Neaton JD, Senguba A. Cigarette smoking as a predictor of death from prostate cancer in 348,874 men screened for the Multiple Risk Factor Intervention Trial. *Am J Epidemiol.* 1996;143:1002–1006.
107. Rodriguez C, Tatham L, Thun M, et al. Smoking and prostate cancer in a large co-hort of adult men. *Am J Epidemiol.* 1997;145:466–475.
108. Couglin SS, Neaton JD, Sengupta A. Cigarette smoking as a predictor of death from prostate cancer in 348,874 men screened for the Multiple Risk Factor Intervention Trial. *Am J Epidemiol.* 1996;143:1002–1006.
109. Cerhan JR, Cantor KP, Williamson K, et al. Cancer mortality among Iowa farmers: recent results, time trends and lifestyle factors. *Cancer Causes Control,* 1998;9:311–319.
110. Buxton JA, Gallagher RP, Le ND, et al. Occupational risk factors for prostate cancer mortality in British Columbia, Canada. *Am J Ind Med.* 1999;35:82–86.
111. Parker AS, Cerhan JR, Putnam SD, et al. A cohort study of farming and risk of prostate cancer in Iowa. *Epidemiology.* 1999;10:452–455.
112. Mills PK, Yang R. Prostate cancer risk in California workers. *J Occup Environ Med.* 2003;45:249–258.
113. Settimi L, Masina A, Andrion A, Alexlson O. Prostate cancer and exposure to pesti-cides in agricultural settings. *Epidemiol.* 2003;104:458–461.
114. Zeegers MP, Friesma IH, Goldbohm RA, van den Brandt PA. A prospective study of occupation and prostate cancer risk. *J Occup Environ Med.* 2004;46:271–279.
115. Hsing AW, Reichart JK, Stanczyk FZ. Hormones and prostate cancer: current per-spectives and future directions. *Prostate.* 2002;52:213–235.
116. Gann PH, Hennekens CH, Ma J, et al. Prospective study of sex hormone levels and risk of prostate cancer. *J Natl Cancer Inst.* 1996;88:1118–1126.
117. Hsing AW, Comstock GW. Serological precursors of cancer: serum hormones and the risk of subsequent cancer of the prostate. *Cancer Epidemiol Biomarkers Prev.* 1993;2:27–32.
118. Dorgan JF, Albanes DV, Virtamo J, et al. Relationships of serum androgens and es-trogens to prostate cancer risk: results from a prospective study in Finland. *Cancer Epidemiol Biomarkers Prev.* 1998;7:1069–1074.
119. Stattin P, Soderberg S, Hallmans G, et al. Leptin is associated with increase prostate cancer risk: a nested case-referent study. *J Clin Endocrinol Metab* 2001;86:1341–1345.
120. Hsing AW, Streamson C, Gao Y-T, et al. Serum levels of insulin and leptin in relation to prostate cancer risk: a population-based case-control study in China. *J Natl Cancer Inst.* 2001;93:783–789.

121. Gann PH, Ma J, Hennekens CH, et al. Circulating vitamin D metabolites in relation to subsequent development of prostate cancer. *Cancer Epidemiol Biomarkers Prev.* 1996;5:121–126.

122. Nomura AM, Stemmermann GN, Lee J, et al. Serum vitamin D metabolite levels and the subsequent development of prostate cancer. *Cancer Causes Control.* 1998;9:425–432.

123. Ahonen MH, Tenkanen L, Teppo L, et al. Prostate cancer and prediagnostic serum 25-hydroxyvitamin D levels (Finland). *Cancer Causes Control.* 2000;11:847–852.

124. Braun MM, Helzlouer KJ, Hollis BW, Comstock GW. Prostate cancer and prediagnostic levels of serum vitamin D metabolites. *Cancer Causes Control.* 1995; 6:235–239.

125. Tuohimaa P, Tenkanen L, Ahonen M, et al. Both high and low levels of blood vitamin D are associated with a higher prostate cancer risk: a longitudinal, nested case-control study in the Nordic countries. *Int J Cancer.* 2004;108:104–108.

126. Dennis LK, Dawson DV. Meta-analysis of measures of sexual activity and prostate cancer. *Epidemiol.* 2002;13:72–79.

127. Dillner J, Knekt P, Borman J, et al. Sero-epidemiological association between human-papillomavirus infection and risk of prostate cancer. *Int J Cancer.* 1998;75:564–567.

128. Hisada M, Rabkin CS, Strickler HD, et al. Human papillomavirus antibody and risk of prostate cancer. *JAMA.* 2000;283:340–341.

129. Giovannucci E, Rimm EB, Colditz GA, et al. A prospective study of dietary fat and risk of prostate cancer. *J Natl Cancer Inst.* 1993;85:1571–1579.

130. Fleshner N, Bagnell PS, Klotz L, Venkateswaran A. Dietary fat and prostate cancer. *J Urol.* 2004;17:S19–S24.

131. Klein EA, Thompson IM, Lippmann S, et al. SELECT: the next prostate cancer prevention trial. *J Urol.* 2001;166:1311–1315.

132. Kristal AR. Vitamin A, retinoids and carotenoids as chemopreventive agents for prostate cancer. *J Urol.* 2004;171:S54–S58.

133. Mills PK, Beeson WL, Phillips R, et al. Cohort study of diet, lifestyle, and prostate cancer in Adventist men. *Cancer.* 1989;64:598–604.

134. Giovannucci E, Ascherio A, Rimm EB. Intake of carotenoids and retinol in relation to prostate cancer risk. *J Natl Cancer Inst.* 1995;87:1767–1776.

135. Gann PH, Ma J, Giovannucci E, et al. Lower prostate cancer risk in men with elevated plasma lycopene levels: results of a prospective analysis. *Cancer Res.* 1999;59:1225–1230.

136. Klein EA. Selenium: epidemiology and basic science. *J Urol.* 2004;171:S50–S53.

137. Clark LC, Combs GF, Turnbull BW, et al. Effects of selenium supplementation for cancer prevention in patients with carcinoma of the skin. A randomized control trial. The National Prevention of Cancer Study Group. *JAMA.* 1996;276: 1957–1963.

138. Duffield-Lillico AJ, Dalkin BL, Reid ME, et al. Selenium supplementation, baseline plasma selenium status, and influence on prostate cancer: an analysis of the complete treatment period of the Nutritional Prevention of Cancer Trial. *Br J Urol.* 2003;91:608–612.

139. Duffield-Lillico AJ, Reid ME, Turnbull BW, et al. Baseline characteristics and the effect of selenium supplementation on cancer risk in a randomized clinical trial: a summary report of the Nutritional Prevention of Cancer Trial. *Cancer Epidemiol Biomarkers Prev.* 2002;11:630–639.

140. Yoshizawa K, Willet WC, Morris S, et al. Study of prediagnostic selenium level in toenails and the risk of advanced prostate cancer. *J Natl Cancer Inst.* 1998;90:1219–1224.
141. Nomura AM, Lee J, Stemmermann GN. Serum selenium and subsequent risk of prostate cancer. *Cancer Epidemiol Biomarkers Prev.* 2000;9:883–887.
142. Vogt TM, Ziegler RG, Graubard BI, et al. Serum selenium and risks of prostate cancer in US blacks and whites. *Int J Cancer.* 2003;103:664-670.
143. Brooks JD, Metter EJ, Chan DW, et al. Plasma selenium level before diagnosis and the risk of prostate cancer development. *J Urol.* 2001;166:2034–2038.
144. Venkateswaran V, Klotz LH, Fleshner NE. Selenium modulation of cell proliferation and cell cycle biomarkers in human prostate cancer cell lines. *Cancer Res.* 2002;62:2540–2545.
145. Bhamre S, Whitin JC, Cohen HJ. Selenomethionine does not affect PSA secretion independent of its effect on LNCaP cell growth. *Prostate.* 2003;54:315–321.
146. Gasparian AV, Yao YJ, Lu J, et al. Selenium compounds inhibit I kappa B kinase (IKK) and nuclear factor-kappa B (NF-kappa B) in prostate cancer cells. *Mol Cancer Ther.* 2002;1:1079–1087.
147. Wang Z, Jiang C, Lu J. Induction of caspase-mediated apoptosis and cell-cycle G1 arrest by selenium metabolite methylselenol. *Mol Carcinogen.* 2002;34:113–120.
148. Bylund A, Zhang JX, Bergh A, et al. Rye bran and soy protein delay growth and increase apoptosis in human LNCap prostate adenocarcinoma in nude mice. *Prostate.* 2000;42:304–314.
149. Zhou JR, Gugger ET, Tanaka T, et al. Soybeans phytochemicals inhibit the growth of transplantable human prostate carcinoma and tumor angiogenesis in mice. *J Nutr.* 1999;129:1628–1635.
150. Mentor-Marcel R, Lamartiniere CA, Eltoum IE, et al. Genistein in the diet reduces the incidence of poorly differentiated prostatic adenocarcinoma in transgenic mice (TRAMP). *Cancer Res.* 2001;61:6777–6782.
151. Davis JN, Singh B, Bhuiyan M, Sakar FH. Genistein-induced upregulation of p21WAF1, downregulation of cyclin B, and induction of apoptosis in prostate cancer cells. *Nutr Cancer.* 1998;32:123–131.
152. Dalu A, Haskell JF, Coward L, Lamartiniere CA. Genistein, a component of soy, inhibits the expression of the EGF, and ERB2/Neu receptors in the rat dorsolateral prostate. *Prostate.* 1998;37:36–43.
153. Evans BA, Griffiths K, Morton MS. Inhibition of 5 alpha-reductase in genital skin fibro-blasts and prostate tissue by dietary lignans and isoflavonoids. *J Endocrinol.* 1995 147:295–302.
154. Jacobsen BK, Knutsen SF, Fraser GE. Does high soy milk intake reduce prostate cancer incidence? The Adventist Health Study (United States). *Cancer Causes Control.* 1998;9:553–557.
155. Lee, MM, Gomez SL, Chang JS, et al. Soy and isoflavone consumption in relation to prostate cancer risk in China. *Cancer Epidemiol Biomarkers Prev.* 2003;12: 665–668.
156. Sonoda T, Nagata Y, Mori M, et al. A case-control study of diet and prostate cancer in Japan: possible protective effect of traditional Japanese diet. *Cancer Sci.* 2004;95:238–242.
157. Gupta S, Hastak K, Ahmad N, et al. Inhibition of prostate carcinogenesis in TRAMP mice by oral infusion of green tea polyphenols. *Proc Natl Acad Sci USA.* 2001;98:10350–10355.

158. Wang SI, Mukhtar H. Gene expression in profile in human prostate LNCaP cancer cells by (–) epigallocatechin-3-gallate. *Cancer Lett.* 2002;182:43–51.
159. Kazi A, Smith DM, Zhong Q, Dou QP. Inhibition of bcl-x(1) phosphorlyation by tea polyphenols or epigallocatechin-3-gallate is associated with prostate cancer apoptosis. *Mol Pharmacol.* 2002;62:765–771.
160. Ren F, Zhang S, Mitchell SH, et al. Tea polyphenols down-regulate the expression of the androgen receptor in the LNCaP prostate cancer cells. *Oncogene.* 2000;19:1924–1932.
161. Jian L, Xie LP, Lee AH, Binns CW. Protective effect of green tea against prostate cancer: a case-control study in southeast China. *Int J Cancer.* 2004;108:130–135.
162. McConnell JD, Roehrborn CG, Baustista O, et al. The long-term effect of doxazosin, finasteride, and combination therapy on clinical progression of benign prostatic hypertrophy. *N Engl J Med.* 2003;349:2387–2398.
163. Thompson IM, Goodman PJ, Tangen C, et al. The influence of finasteride on the development of prostate cancer, *N Engl J Med.* 2003;349:215–224.
164. Djavan B, Zlotta A, Schulman C, et al. Chemoprevention studies of prostate cancer. *J Urol.* 2004;171:S10–S13.
165. Steiner MS, Raghow S, Neubauer BL. Selective estrogen receptor modulators for the chemoprevention of prostate cancer. *Urology.* 2001;57:68–72.
166. Barqawi A, Thompson IM, Crawford ED. Prostate cancer chemoprevention: an overview of United States trials. *J Urol.* 2004;171:S5–S8.
167. Heinonen OP, Albanes D, Virtamo J, et al. Prostate cancer and supplementation with alpha-tocopherol and beta-carotene: incidence and mortality in a controlled trial. *J Natl Cancer Inst.* 1998;90:440–446.
168. Christen WG, Gaziano J, Hennekens CH. Design of Physicians' Health Study II-a randomized trial of beta-carotene, vitamins E and C, and multivitamins, in prevention of cancer, cardiovascular disease, and eye disease, and review of completed trials. *Ann Epidemiol.* 2000;10:125–134.
169. Clark LC, Dalkin B, Krongad A, et al. Decreased incidence of prostate cancer with selenium supplementation: results of a double-blind cancer prevention trial. *Br J Urol.* 1998;81:730–734.
170. Smith RA, Cokkinides V, Erye HJ. American Cancer Society Guidelines for the Early Detection of Cancer, 2005. *Ca Cancer J Clin.* 2005;55:31–44.

Chapter 2

Screening and Early Detection

INTRODUCTION[1, 2]

No consensus on who should be screened. Recommendations range from no screening to screening all men.

THE CONTROVERSY OVER SCREENING[3-7]

Use of prostate-specific antigen (PSA) has resulted in the increased diagnosis of early-stage potentially significant prostate cancers.

Groups advocating screening include[1, 8]
- American Cancer Society, American Urologic Association, American College of Radiology, the Prostate Education Council, National Comprehensive Cancer Network (NCCN)

Groups not advocating screening at this time include[9]
- National Cancer Institute, US Preventive Services Task Force, Canadian Task Force on the Periodic Health Examination, Centers for Disease Control and Prevention, American Academy of Family Physicians, American College of Preventive Medicine

Research supporting screening
- Labrie et al.[10]—Prospective randomized trial comparing screening with digital rectal examination (DRE) and PSA the first year of screening followed by PSA tests the following years versus no screening. Beneficial effect of screening demonstrated in this study with fewer prostate cancer-related deaths in the screened group. Additional research on screening is needed.

HIGH RISK FACTOR AND CONTRIBUTING FACTORS[11-23]

Age

- Incidence of prostate cancer increases with age, particularly after age 50

Family History

- Familial cancer—Family cluster of prostate cancer occurs. Father, brother, or son with prostate cancer increases risk of individual family member.
- Positive family history present in approximately 25% of patients.
- Hereditary factors account for approximately 10% of prostate cancers.

Race

- Native Americans—Lowest incidence rate with poorest survival for localized or regional disease
- African-Americans—Highest prostate cancer rate with highest mortality rate in the world

Diet

Dietary fat
- Strong environmental factor for prostate cancer-high fat diets high in saturated fats

- Countries (Asian) with low rates of prostate cancer consume lower fat diets. Immigration to United States increases prostate cancer risk in first generation Chinese-Americans and Japanese-Americans.

Selenium
  - Essential trace nutrient with antioxidant properties
  - Reduces prostate cancer incidence
  - Clinical trials underway in patients with prostatic intraepithelial neoplasia to assess effect of selenium on prostate cancer development

Vitamins
  - Vitamin E may reduce mortality rates.
  - Vitamin E and selenium being studied in Selenium and Vitamin E Cancer Prevention Trial (SELECT).

Lycopene
  - A carotenoid found in processed and cooked tomatoes may reduce risk of prostate cancer.

Testosterone levels
  - Increased testosterone levels may be associated with an increased risk of prostate cancer in African-Americans.
  - Levels are about 15% higher in African-Americans.
  - Dihydrotestosterone-testosterone ratios are highest in African-Americans.

WHO SHOULD BE SCREENED[8, 24, 25]

American Cancer Society screening guidelines
  - Discussion between the patient and the physician regarding the significance of screening outcomes, implications, risks, and benefits of screening is important before undergoing the procedures.
  - Screening includes annual DRE and PSA beginning at age 50 (see **Table 2–1**).

NCCN screening guidelines
  - Released in 2004
  - Recommend screening all men age $\geq$ 50 with at least a 10-year expected survival time

TABLE 2–1 American Cancer Society Screening Guidelines

Population	DRE	PSA
Asymptomatic men with no high-risk factors and at least a 10-year life expectancy	Annually after age 50	Annually after age 50
Men with high-risk factors • African-American • Two or more first-degree relatives with prostate cancer	Annually before age 50 (at approximately age 45)	Annually before age 50 (at approximately age 45)

DRE, digital rectal examination, PSA, prostate-specific antigen.
Source: Waldman AR. Screening and early detection. In: Held-Warmkessel, J., ed. *Contemporary Issues in Prostate Cancer: A Nursing Perspective* (2nd ed). Jones and Bartlett Publishers, 2006, 44–59. Reprinted with permission by Jones and Bartlett Publishers.

- Recommend biopsy if PSA > 2.5 ng/mL
- African-Americans should be screened starting age 45 or earlier (at age 40 for PSA > 0.5 ng/mL and positive family history).
- cPSA assay cutoff value of 3.0 mg/mL

FACTORS INFLUENCING SCREENING FOR CANCER[26-32]

- Physician recommendation
- Family or friend diagnosis with prostate cancer
- Scheduled appointment with reminder
- Encouragement by role model of same ethnic group
- Personalized education
- Community-based annual screenings led by a community leader
- Community-based education

BARRIERS TO SCREENING[33-36]

- Beliefs and practices of ethnic or cultural groups
- Health concepts of cultural groups
- Fear of diagnostic studies, cancer diagnosis, treatment-related side effects
- Lack of insurance
- Lack of access to health care

SCREENING TOOLS[37-39]

Digital rectal examination
- Performed in one of three possible positions
- Posterior and lateral aspects of gland palpated during examination
- Anterior tumors cannot be felt during DRE.
- Small tumors may not be detected by DRE.
- Examiner assesses gland for abnormal areas—induration, asymmetry, nodularity
- When used as a single screening modality, 40% of tumors are not found.

Prostate-specific antigen[8, 39-51]
- Found in prostate gland epithelial cells
- Level increases with increased gland size; may be from benign or malignant causes
- Levels increase with ejaculation (for 48 hours) and with manipulation of the gland such as cystoscopy, prostate biopsy, or transurethral resection of the prostate (TURP) (see **Table 2–2**). With these procedures, PSA levels may remain elevated for 4 weeks and should wait 6 weeks for PSA levels to be drawn after a biopsy or TURP.
- Physicians often prefer to obtain a PSA specimen prior to DRE even though evidence demonstrating that DRE increased PSA levels is not significant.
- Food and Drug Administration approved PSA for use with DRE in evaluating men ≥ 50 years old for prostate cancer.
- Patients should use the same laboratory for follow-up PSA levels to reduce variability in test results due to different PSA tests used by different laboratories.
- Home use kits are available.
- Normal PSA level is 0.0–4.0 ng/mL.

Age-related prostate-specific antigen
- May be more sensitive for patients < 60 with an increased potential for finding localized disease

- May be more specific for patients > 60 with a reduced need for unnecessary biopsies
- May not be useful for African-American men who have higher PSA levels and levels that occur over a wider range

Age- and race-specific reference ranges
- Vary based on reference used; see **Tables 2–3** and **2–4**
- Methods to improve PSA specificity from the American Urologic Association Best Practice Task Force include age-adjusted PSA, free-to-total PSA, and PSA density.[51]

Uses of transrectal ultrasound (TRUS)[52]
- Needle biopsy of the prostate
- A screening adjunct when abnormality found on DRE or PSA is elevated
- Measuring gland size and shape, volume, and density

COST VERSUS BENEFIT OF EARLY DETECTION[53]

- Cost includes amount for screening, follow-up testing, treatment, and management of treatment-related complications.
- Benefit may be greatest for men in their 50s and 60s.

TABLE 2–2 Factors Affecting PSA

Increase	Decrease
Acute prostatitis	Finasteride
Acute urinary retention	Bedrest
Benign prostatic hyperplasia (BPH)	Saw palmetto
Ejaculation (up to 48 hours after)	Other agents that reduce 5-α-reductase
Prostate biopsy	
TRUS-guided biopsy	

PSA, prostate-specific antigen; TRUS, transrectal ultrasonography.

Adapted from Oesterling et al.,[41] Crawford et al.,[42] Yuan et al.,[43] and Oesterling and Moyad.[44]

Source: Waldman, AR. Screening and early detection. In: Held-Warmkessel, J., ed. *Contemporary Issues in Prostate Cancer: A Nursing Perspective* (2nd ed). Jones and Bartlett Publishers, 2006, 44–59. Reprinted with permission by Jones and Bartlett Publishers.

TABLE 2–3 Age-Specific Reference Ranges for the PSA Test According to Race

Age (yr)	Caucasians	African-Americans
40–49	0–2.5	0–2.0
50–59	0–3.5	0–4.0
60–69	0–3.5	0–4.5
70–79	0–3.5	0–5.5

PSA, prostate-specific antigen.

Source: Adapted 1999 with permission from Morgan TO, Jacobsen SJ, McCarthy WF, et al. Age-specific reference ranges for serum prostate-specific antigen in black men. *N Engl J Med.* 1996;335:304–310. Copyright © 1996 Massachusetts Medical Society. All rights reserved. Used with permission.

TABLE 2–4 Age-Specific Reference Ranges for Serum PSA

	Reference Range		
	Asians	African-Americans	Whites
40–49 yr	0–2.0 ng/mg	0–2.0 ng/mL	0–2.5 ng/mL
50–59 yr	0–3.0 ng/mg	0–4.0 ng/mL	0–3.5 ng/mL
60–69 yr	0–4.0 ng/mL	0–4.5 ng/mL	0–4.5 ng/mL
70–79 yr	0–5.0 ng/mL	0–5.5 ng/mL	0–6.5 ng/mL

Source: PSA Best Practice Policy from the American Urological Association (AUA). *Oncology.* 2000;14:267–286. Used with permission from The Oncology Group, a division of CMP Healthcare Media, Manhasset, New York, Copyright 2000.

References

1. Hoffman RM, Blume MD, Gilliland F. Prostate-specific antigen testing practices and outcomes. *J Gen Intern Med.* 1998;13:106–110.
2. U.S. Preventive Services Task Force. *U.S. Preventive Services Task Force Guide to Clinical Preventive Services.* Baltimore, Md: Williams & Wilkins; 1996.
3. Lodding P, Aus G, Bergdahl R, et al. Characteristics of screening detected prostate cancer in men 50 to 66 years old with 3 to 4 ng/mL prostate specific antigen. *J Urol.* 1998;159:899–903.
4. Mettlin CJ, Murphy GP, Babaian RJ, et al. Observations on the early detection of prostate cancer from the American Cancer Society National Prostate Cancer Detection Project. *Cancer.* 1997;80:1814–1817.
5. Newcomer LM, Stanford JL, Blunenstein BA, Brawer MK. Temporal trends in rates of prostate cancer: declining incidence of advanced stage disease, 1974–1994. *J Urol.* 1997;158:1427–1430.
6. Reissigl A, Horninger W, Fink K, et al. Prostate carcinoma screening in the county of Tyrol, Austria: experience and results. *Cancer.* 1997;80:1818–1829.
7. Smith DS, Humphrey PA, Catalona WJ. The early detection of prostate carcinoma with prostate specific antigen. *Cancer.* 1997;80:1852–1856.
8. National Comprehensive Cancer Network. Practice Guidelines in Oncology—Prostate cancer early detection. Available at: http://www.nccn.com/physician_gls/PDF _prostate.pdf. Accessed February 19, 2005.
9. Ferrini R, Woolf S. Screening for prostate cancer in American men. American College of Preventive Medicine Practice Policy Statement. Available at: http://www .acpm.org/prostate.htm. Accessed February 19, 2005.
10. Labrie F, Dupont A, Candas B, et al. Decrease of prostate cancer death by screening: first data from the Quebec prospective and randomized study [abstract 4]. *Proc Am Soc Clin Oncol.* 1998;17:2a.
11. Lind J. Nursing care of the client with cancer of the urinary system. In: Itano JK, Taoka KN, eds. *Core Curriculum for Oncology Nursing.* 3rd ed. Philadelphia, Pa: WB Saunders; 1998:421–447.
12. Gronberg H, Damber L, Damber JE. Familial prostate cancer in Sweden. A nationwide register cohort study. *Cancer.* 1996;77:138–143.
13. Whittemore AS, Wu AH, Kolonel LN, et al. Family history and prostate cancer risk in black, white, and Asian men in the United States and Canada. *Am J Epidemiol.* 1995;121:732–740.

14. Walsh PC, Partin AW. Family history facilitates the early diagnosis of prostate carcinoma. *Cancer.* 1997;80:1871–1874.

15. Carter BS, Beaty TH, Steinberg GD, et al. Mendelian inheritance of familial prostate cancer. *Proc Natl Acad Sci USA.* 1992;89:3367–3371.

16. National Cancer Institute. Prostate cancer: racial/ethnic patterns. Available at: http://www.seer.cancer.gov. Accessed February 19, 2005.

17. Wingo P, Bolden S, Tong T, et al. Cancer statistics for African-Americans. *CA Cancer J Clin.* 1996;46:113–117.

18. Brosman SA, Moyad M. Prostate cancer: nutrition. 2004. Available at: http://www.emedicine.com/med/topics3100.htm. Accessed February 19, 2005.

19. Groenwald SL, Frogge MH, Goodman M, Yarbro CH, eds. *Comprehensive Cancer Nursing Review.* Sudbury, Mass: Jones and Bartlett; 1998:552.

20. Clark LD, Dalkin B, Krongard A. Decreased incidence of prostate cancer with selenium supplementation: results of a double-blind cancer prevention trial. *Br J Urol.* 1998;5:730–734.

21. National Cancer Institute. Clinical trials. Available at: http://cancer.gov Clinical Trials(PDQ®). February 19, 2005.

22. National Cancer Institute SELECT Trial. Available at: http://cancer.gov/clinicaltrial/digestpage/SELECT. Accessed February 19, 2005.

23. Wu AH, Whittemore AS, Kolonel LN. Serum androgens and sex hormone—binding globulins in relation to lifestyle factors in older African-Americans, white, and Asian men in the United States and Canada. *Cancer Epidemiol Biomarkers Prev.* 1995;4:735–741.

24. National Cancer Institute. Report from large NCI study suggests PSA testing could be done at longer intervals for men who choose to test. 2002. Available at: http://www.cancer.gov/prevention/plco/index.html. Accessed February 19, 2005.

25. American Cancer Society. ACS cancer detection guidelines. Available at: http://www.cancer.org/docroot/ContentPED_2_3X_ACS_Cancer_Detection_Guidelines_36.asp?sitearea=PED. February 19, 2005.

26. McKee JM. Cue to action in prostate cancer screening. *Oncol Nurs Forum.* 1994;21:1171–1176.

27. Steele CB, Miller DS, Maylahn C, et al. Knowledge, attitudes, and screening practices among older men regarding prostate cancer. *Am J Public Health.* 2000;90:1595–1600.

28. Williams E, Vessey M. Randomized trial of two strategies offering women mobile screening for breast cancer. *BMJ.* 1989;299:158–159.

29. Wilson A, Leemings A. Cervical cytology: a comparison of two call systems. *BMJ.* 1987;295:181–182.

30. Wolosin R. Effect of appointment scheduling and reminder post cards on adherence to mammography recommendations. *J Fam Pract.* 1990;30:542–547.

31. Weinrich SP, Boyd MD, Weinrich M, et al. Increasing prostate cancer screening in African American men with peer-educator and client-navigator interventions. *J Cancer Educ.* 1998;13:213–219.

32. Waldman AR, Starr S, Tester W, et al. Awareness of prostate cancer in African American men and its influence on screening health behaviors. Poster presentation at the American Public Health Association Annual Meeting, Boston, Mass. November 13, 2002.

33. Centers for Medicare and Medicaid Services. "Stay healthy: Overview. 2004. Available at: http://www.medicare.gov/Health/Overview.asp. February 19, 2005.

34. Kagawa-Singer M. Addressing issues for early detection and screening in ethnic populations. *Oncol Nurs Forum*. 1997;24:1705–1714.

35. Braithwaite RL. Health status of black men. In: Braithwaite RL, Taylor SE, eds. *Health Issues in the Black Community*. San Francisco, Calif: Jossey-Bass Publisher; 2001:62–80.

36. Powell IJ. Early detection issues of prostate cancer in African American men. *In Vivo*. 1994;8:451–452.

37. Littrup PJ, Lee F, Mettlin C. Prostate cancer screening: current trends and future implications. *CA Cancer J Clin*. 1992;42:198–211.

38. Catalona WJ, Richie JP, Ahmann FR, et al. Comparison of digital rectal examinations and serum prostate specific antigen in the early detection of prostate cancer: results of a multicentered clinical trial of 6,630 men. *J Urol*. 1994;1551:1283–1290.

39. Coley CM, Barry MJ, Mulley AG. Screening for prostate cancer. *Ann Intern Med*. 1997;126:480–484.

40. Gelfand DE, Parzuchowski J, Cort M, Powell I. Digital rectal examinations and prostate cancer screening: attitudes of African American men. *Oncol Nurs Forum*. 1995;22:1253–1255.

41. Oesterling JE, Rice DC, Glenski WJ, Bergstralh EJ. Effect of cystoscopy, prostate biopsy, and transurethral resection of prostate on serum prostate-specific antigen concentration. *Urology*. 1993:42:276–282.

42. Crawford ED, Schutz MJ, Clejan S, et al. The effect of digital rectal examination on prostate-specific antigen levels. *JAMA*. 1992;267:2227–2228.

43. Yuan JJ, Copen DE, Petros JA, et al. Effects of rectal examination, prostatic massage, ultrasonography and needle biopsy on serum prostate specific antigen levels. *J Urol*. 1992;147:810–814.

44. Oesterling JE, Moyad MA. *The ABCs of Prostate Cancer: The Book That Could Save Your Life*. Lanham, Md: Madison Books; 1997:40,49.

45. Diagnostic Products Corporation. FDA approves DPC's total immunoreactive PSA assays for prostate cancer detection. Available at: http://www.dpcweb.cm/documents/new&views/summer01/fda_approval/html. Accessed February 19, 2005.

46. Oesterling JE, Jacobsen SJ, Chute CG, et al. Serum prostate-specific antigen in a community-based population of healthy men: establishment of age-specific reference ranges. *JAMA*. 1993;270: 860–864.

47. Oesterling JE. Using prostate-specific antigen to eliminate unnecessary diagnostic tests: significant worldwide economic implications. *Urology*. 1995;46(3 suppl A):26–33.

48. Morgan TO, Jacobsen SJ, McCarthy WF, et al. Age-specific reference ranges for serum prostate-specific antigen in black men. *N Engl J Med*. 1996;335:304–310.

49. Catalona WJ, Smith DS, Ornstein DK. Prostate cancer detection in men with serum PSA concentrations of 2.6 to 4.0 ng/mL and benign prostate examination: Enhancement of specificity with free PSA measurements. *JAMA*. 1997;277:1452–1455.

50. American Urological Association. PSA Best Practice Policy Task Force. Prostate-Specific Antigen (PSA) Best Practice Policy. *Oncology*. 2000;14:267–286.

51. DeAntoni EP. Age-specific reference ranges for PSA in the detection of prostate cancer. *Oncology*. 1997;11:475–485.

52. Olson MC, Posniak HV, Fisher SG, et al. Directed and random biopsies of the prostate: indications based on combined results of transrectal sonography and prostate-specific antigen density determinations. *Am J Roentgenol*. 1994;163: 1407–1411.

53. Coley CM, Barry MJ, Fleming C, et al. Early detection of prostate cancer. Part II: Estimating the risks, benefits, and costs. *Ann Intern Med*. 1997;126:468–479.

Part II
Disease Assessment

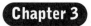

Cellular Characteristics, Pathophysiology, and Disease Manifestations

CARCINOGENESIS AND PATHOLOGY

Carcinogenesis[1, 2]

- Development of cancer

Stages of carcinogenesis
Initiation
- Carcinogen-induced DNA damage resulting in either cellular repair or cellular damage (mutation)

Promotion
- Reversible or irreversible carcinogen-induced cell injury

Progression
- Accumulation of additional cellular damage; cell may behave in a malignant manner.

Invasion
Angiogenesis
Growth factor stimulation
Metastases

Oncogenes
- Genes that promote cancer growth; affected by carcinogens
- Prostate gland may contain normal, premalignant, and malignant cells.
- Cells accumulate multiple changes over time.

Prostatic Intraepithelial Neoplasia (PIN)[1, 3–16]

- Premalignant lesion of the prostate. Cells not completely transformed to a malignant state
- Prostate cancer precursor
- Has many of the same cell changes as cancer with loss of differentiation and regulatory control
- Multifocal
- Ability to spread via ducts
- Usually located in peripheral zone but also found in transitional zone

PIN divided into low-grade PIN and high-grade PIN
- Low-grade PIN is less likely to be associated with the development of prostate cancer.
- High-grade PIN is associated with the development of prostate cancer.
- High-grade PIN is the presence of cellular abnormalities seen in cancer, such as abnormal cell structure.
- PIN may be present up to 10 years before cancer diagnosis.
- Incidence of PIN may increase with aging.

- Extent of PIN may increase with aging.
- The more dysplastic the cells, the greater the risk of cancer.
- High-grade PIN is often associated with cancer on biopsy specimens.

The presence of high-grade PIN
- Aids in the prediction of a prostate cancer diagnosis
- Repeat biopsies may be necessary to accurately diagnose prostate cancer.
- Additional diagnostic studies to assess for the presence of prostate cancer may be needed.
- Without evidence of cancer, repeat biopsies are recommended every 3–6 months for 2 years, and then yearly.
- Patient preference for therapy, patient's age, and patient's medical condition may play a role in follow-up decisions.
- PIN may be more predictive of cancer in African-American males.
- PIN may be more predictive of cancer in males with an abnormal prostate-specific antigen (PSA) level.
- The natural history of PIN requires ongoing research.
- Presently unable to determine if PIN will progress, remain stable, or regress.
- PIN may be more predictive of cancer if multifocal on initial biopsy.

Atypical Adenomatous Hyperplasia (AAH)[17–18]

- Status as a premalignant lesion not yet confirmed
- Found in transitional zone most frequently.

PATHOPHYSIOLOGY OF PROSTATE CANCER[3, 19, 20]

Majority of Tumors Are Adenocarcinomas

- Embryonic urogenital sinus epithelium is the cell of origin.

Other Cell Types of Epithelial Origin

- Pure ductal and mucinous adenocarcinomas, small cell tumors, transitional cell carcinoma, carcinoma in situ (includes intraepithelial neoplasia)

Carcinosarcoma
Nonepithelial Neoplasms

- Malignant mesenchymal tumors, lymphomas (metastatic site)

Germ Cell Tumors
Secondary Tumors

- Metastatic germ cell tumors; metastatic tumors from other pelvic cancers such as cancers of the bladder, urethra, colon, rectum, or anus; malignant lymphoma, bone or soft tissue sarcomas, alimentary tract carcinoma, or leukemia

---

GRADING AND PROGNOSTIC INDICATORS OF PROSTATE CANCER[7, 19–26]

Grading

- Amount of histologic change in cellular characteristics and cellular architecture between normal cells and malignant cells is used to describe a tumor's potential behavior.

Gleason Grading System

- Commonly used to describe prostate cancer histology and cellular architecture

Five histologic patterns, grades 1 to 5
- Grade 1 tumors are well differentiated
- Grade 5 tumors are poorly differentiated
- Many tumors exhibit two types of histologic pattern
- Each tumor is given two grades: one grade is assigned to the most common tumor pattern present in the specimen, and a second grade is given to the second most common tumor pattern present in the specimen. The grades are added to give a total possible score of 2–10.

Prognostic Indicators

Tumor grade
- Gleason scores of 7–10 predict higher risk of nodal metastases and decreased survival
- High-grade tumors have more neuroendocrine tumor cells and more neovascularization

Tumor volume
- Low Gleason grade (1–2) tumors are usually under 1 cc in size
- High Gleason grade (4–5) tumors are usually over 1 cc in size

Clinical stage
Tumor location
- Transition zone tumors are less aggressive than those in the peripheral zone

Serum PSA
- Higher grade tumors (Gleason score 7 or higher) are associated with elevated serum PSA (> 10 ng/mL)

Capsular penetration and spread
- Associated with Gleason score > 7
- PSA > 8 indicates greater risk of seminal vesicle spread, lymph node metastasis, and bone metastasis

Patient age
Patient's health status
Grade, PSA, stage, tumor location, and elevated prostatic acid phosphatase (PAP) all correlate.
Flow cytometry

FACTORS FOR TUMOR DEVELOPMENT, PROGRESSION, AND METASTASIS[1, 3, 19–21, 27-30]

Natural History

- Increasing incidence with aging
- Tumor location in peripheral zone
- Histologic and biochemical changes occur
- Grade associated with spread
- Spreads along tissue planes
- Spreads to lymph nodes and bone
- Androgen dependent

Hereditary or Genetic Factors

- Caused by multiple factors—genetic, hormonal, environmental—resulting in altered genetic function

- Loss of tumor-suppressor genes
- Presence of oncogenes promoting tumor growth
- Presence of heritable genetic factor plus environmental carcinogens
- Loss of metastatic-suppressor genes, such as wild type p53 gene
- Altered DNA methylation
- Hormonal and environmental factors may also be involved.
- Loss of balance between cell growth and cell death
- Inflammation
- Altered growth factors

Angiogenesis[3, 19, 20, 31–35]

- Process of development of new blood vessel growth by a tumor
- Tumor growth is dependent on the ability to develop a new blood supply. Size of tumor is limited by blood supply.
- Microvessel density may portend disease progression

Two stages of vascular-based disease progression
  Prevascular
- Early in tumor development; little cell growth
  Vascular
- Presence of increased blood vessels and tumor growth
- Process of angiogenesis occurs prior to conversion of the tumor to malignant status and metastases
- Role of VEG-F—regulates angiogenesis

Location of Disease[1, 3, 7, 10, 12, 19]

Important considerations regarding disease location
  Regional distribution of disease
- Peripheral zone: 70–75% of cancers originate in this zone
- Impact on ability to spread locally
- Higher-grade tumors and higher-grade PIN
  Multicentricity of prostate cancer
- Multiple tumors at different sites in the prostate gland each with different specificity including size, malignant biologic potential, and cellular characteristics

Progression of Disease[1, 3, 36]

Routes of growth
  Initial growth
- Along tissue planes in prostate gland, including intraprostatic and periprostatic
- Higher-grade lesions are more aggressive and able to cross tissue planes.
- Peripheral zone lesions spread to periprostatic tissue.
  Extraprostatic spread
- To base of bladder and seminal vesicles
- Perineural invasion
  Pelvic lymph nodes
- Spread to obturator, presacral, hypogastric, common iliac, and inguinal nodes axial skeleton
- By time of death 80% of patients are affected; involvement may include spine, femur, pelvis, ribs, skull, or humerus.
  Metastatic sites
- Lungs
- Liver
- Kidneys

Role of Androgens[27, 37, 38]

Androgens are required for normal prostate structure and function. Normal physiology:

- Testicular production of testosterone
  ↓
- Conversion to dihydrotestosterone (DHT)
  ↓
- Binds to androgen receptors (AR) in prostate
  ↓
- DHT-androgen receptor (AR) complex controls prostate growth genes and cellular apoptosis.
- Adrenal androgens are weaker than androgens of testicular origin but are also converted to DHT.

Prostate cancers are initially androgen sensitive and become androgen independent. Role of androgens in prostate carcinogenesis is unclear. Initial androgen therapy is effective in 70–80% of patients. Androgen independence may be caused by change in AR, change in AR target gene, or change in AR signal. Result is loss of apoptosis.

CLINICAL MANIFESTATIONS[1, 3, 36, 39]

Early Stage Disease

- Often asymptomatic
- If located in transition zone or near the urethra, may result in symptoms of bladder outlet obstruction—frequency, hesitancy, dysuria, slow stream, nocturia, urgency, dribbling, hesitancy, retention, and incontinence.
- Involvement of seminal vesicles may cause hematospermia.
- Involvement of ejaculatory ducts may cause reduced ejaculate volume.
- Involvement of neurovascular bundles may cause impotence.

Advanced Disease

- Bone pain, back pain
- Anemia, pancytopenia
- Weight loss
- Perineal pain
- Leg pain

References

1. Held-Warmkessel J. Prostate cancer. In: Groenwald SL, Frogge MH, Goodman M, Yarbro CH, eds. *Cancer Nursing Principles & Practice*. Sudbury, Mass: Jones and Bartlett; 1997:1334–1354.
2. Volker DL. Carcinogenesis. In: Itano JK, Taoka KN, eds. *ONS Core Curriculum for Oncology Nursing*. 3rd ed. Philadelphia, Pa: WB Saunders; 1998:357–382.
3. Oesterling J, Fuks Z, Lee CT, Scher HI. Cancer of the prostate. In: DeVita VT Jr, Hellman S, Rosenberg SA, eds. *Cancer: Principles & Practice of Oncology*. 5th ed. Philadelphia, Pa: Lippincott-Raven; 1997:1322–1345.
4. Pacelli A, Bostwick DG. Clinical significance of high-grade prostatic intraepithelial neoplasia in transurethral resection specimens. *Urology*. 1997;50:355–359.
5. Wills ML, Hamper UM, Partin AW, Epstein JI. Incidence of high grade prostatic intraepithelial neoplasia in sextant needle biopsy specimens. *Urology*. 1997;49:367–373.

6. Bostwick DG. High grade prostatic intraepithelial neoplasia: the most likely precursor of prostate cancer. *Cancer.* 1995;75(suppl):1823–1836.
7. Haggman MJ, Macoska JA, Wojno KJ, Oesterling JE. The relationship between prostatic intraepithelial neoplasia and prostate cancer: critical issues. *J Urol.* 1997;158:12–22.
8. Brosman SA. Prostatic intraepithelial neoplasia (PIN). eMedicine Clinical Knowledge Base, 2001. Available at: www.emedicine.com. May 16, 2006.
9. Zlotta AR, Raviv G, Schulman CC. Clinical prognostic criteria for later diagnosis of prostate carcinoma in patients with initial isolated prostatic intraepithelial neoplasia. *Eur Urol.* 1996;30:249–255.
10. Bostwick DG, Pacelli A, Lopez-Beltran A. Molecular biology of prostatic intraepithelial neoplasia. *Prostate.* 1996;29:117–134.
11. Anonymous. Prostatic intraepithelial neoplasia: significance and correlation with prostate-specific antigen and transrectal ultrasound. Proceedings of a workshop of the National Prostate Cancer Detection Project, March 13, 1989. Bethesda, Md. *Urology.* 1989;34(suppl):2.
12. Bostwick DG. Progression of prostatic intraepithelial neoplasia to early invasive adenocarcinoma. *Eur Urol.* 1996;30:145–152.
13. Bostwick DG, Qian I, Frankel K. The incidence of high grade prostatic intraepithelial neoplasia in needle biopsies. *J Urol.* 1995;154:1791–1794.
14. Davidson D, Bostwick DG, Qian I, et al. Prostatic intraepithelial neoplasia is a risk factor for adenocarcinoma: predictive accuracy in needle biopsies. *J Urol.* 1996; 154:1295–1299.
15. Berner A, Skjorten FJ, Fossa SD. Follow-up of prostatic intraepithelial neoplasia. *Eur Urol.* 1996;30:256–260.
16. Roscigno M, Scattoni V, Freschi M, et al. Monofocal and plurifocal high grade prostatic intraepithelial neoplasia on extended prostate biopsies: factors predicting cancer detection on extended repeat biopsy. *Urology.* 2004;63:1105–1110.
17. Bostwick DG. Prospective origins of prostate carcinoma: prostatic intraepithelial neoplasia and atypical adenomatous hyperplasia. *Cancer.* 1996;78:330–336.
18. Cheng L, Shan A, Cheville JC, et al. Atypical adenomatous hyperplasia of the prostate: a premalignant lesion. *Cancer Res.* 1998;58:389–391.
19. Kozlowski JM, Grayhack JT. Carcinoma of the prostate. In: Gillenwater JY, Grayhack JT, Howard SS, Duckett JW, eds. *Adult and Pediatric Urology.* 3rd ed. St. Louis, Mo: CV Mosby; 1996:1575–1713.
20. Bostwick DG. Evaluating prostate needle biopsy: therapeutic and prognostic importance. *CA Cancer J Clin.* 1997;47:297–319.
21. Newman J. Epidemiology, diagnosis and treatment of prostate cancer. *Radiol Technol.* 1996;68:39–68.
22. Bostwick DG. Grading prostate cancer. *Am J Clin Pathol.* 1994;102:538–556.
23. Debes JD, Tindall DJ. Mechanisms of androgen-refractory prostate cancer. *N Engl J Med.* 2004;351:1488–1490.
24. Grobholz R, Bohrer MH, Siefsmund M, et al. Correlation between neovascularization and neuroendocrine differentiation in prostatic carcinoma. *Pathol Res Pract.* 2000;196:277–284.
25. Stenman UH. Prostate specific antigen, clinical use and staging: an overview. *Br J Urol.* 1997;79:53–60.
26. Dattoli M, Wallner K, True L, et al. Prognostic role of serum prostatic acid phosphatase for 103-Pd based radiation for prostatic carcinoma. *Int J Radiat Oncol Biol Phys.* 1999;45:853–856.

27. Boulikas T. Gene therapy of prostate cancer: p53, suicidal genes, and other targets. *Anticancer Res.* 1997;17:1471–1506.
28. Denmeade SR, Lin XS, Isaacs JT. Role of programmed (apoptotic) cell death during the progression and therapy for prostate cancer. *Prostate.* 1996;23:251–265.
29. Humphrey PA, Swanson PE. Immunoreactive p53 protein in high-grade prostatic intraepithelial neoplasia. *Pathol Res Pract.* 1995;191:881–887.
30. De Marzo AM, DeWeese TL, Platz EA, et al. Pathological and molecular mechanisms of prostate carcinogenesis: implications for diagnosis, detection, prevention and treatment. *J Cell Biochem.* 2004;91:459–477.
31. Siegal JA, Yu E, Brawer MK. Topography of neovascularity in human prostate carcinoma. *Cancer.* 1995;75:2545–2551.
32. Folkman J, Watson K, Ingber D, Hanahan D. Introduction of angiogenesis during the transition from hyperplasia to neoplasia. *Nature.* 1989;339:58–61.
33. Ferrer FA, Miller LJ, Andrawis RI, et al. Angiogenesis and prostate cancer: in vivo and in vitro expression of angiogenesis factors by prostate cancer cells. *Urology.* 1998;51:161–167.
34. Walsh K, Sriprasad S, Hopster D, et al. Distribution of vascular endothelial growth factor (VEGF) in prostate disease. *Prostate Cancer Prostatic Dis.* 2002;5:119–122.
35. Ferrara, N Vascular endothelial growth factor as a target for anticancer therapy. *Oncologist.* 2004;9(suppl):2–10.
36. McGinnis DE, Gomella LG. Tumors of the prostate. In: Babnson RR, ed. *Management of Urologic Disorders.* London, UK: Wolfe; 1994:5.2–5.31.
37. Dorkin TJ, Neal DE. Basic science aspects of prostate cancer. *Semin Cancer Biol.* 1997;8:21–27.
38. Griffiths K, Morton MS, Nicholson RI. Androgens, androgen receptors, antiandrogens and the treatment of prostate cancer. *Eur Urol.* 1997;32:24–40.
39. American Cancer Society. *Cancer Facts & Figures.* Atlanta, Ga: ACS; 2004.

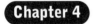

Assessment and Diagnosis

CLINICAL PRESENTATION[1-3]

Localized Disease

- Many newly diagnosed patients present at this stage due to PSA elevation or an abnormal DRE

Symptoms may or may not be present and may include
Asymptomatic
- Related to tumor location in peripheral areas of gland in 68% of patients
Lower urinary tract obstructive or irritative voiding symptoms
- Hesitancy, reduced urinary stream force, intermittency, frequency, and postvoid dribbling due to urethral blockage from enlarging prostate gland. See **Table 4–1** for comparison of obstructive and irritative voiding symptoms.

Rare presenting symptoms
- Ejaculatory duct blockage
- Reduced ejaculate volume; hematospermia
- Invasion of neurovascular bundle
- Impotence

Local invasion of prostatic urethra/bladder base
Hematuria (rare)

Metastatic Disease

Bone metastases, osteoblastic lesions
- Bone pain, spinal cord compression, pancytopenia, anemia

Pelvic or inguinal lymph node metastases
- Lower extremity edema
- Scrotal edema

Ureteral obstruction with hydronephrosis
- Renal failure

TABLE 4–1 Voiding Symptoms

Obstructive Symptoms	Irritative Symptoms
- Hesitancy	- Frequency
- Decreased urinary stream force	- Nocturia
- Intermittent voiding	- Urgency
	- Urge incontinence

Source: Roethke SK. Initial assessment and diagnosis. In: Held-Warmkessel, J., ed. *Contemporary Issues in Prostate Cancer: A Nursing Perspective* (2nd ed). Jones and Bartlett Publishers, 2006, 79–106. Reprinted with permission by Jones and Bartlett Publishers.

Visceral metastases (lung, liver, bladder, adrenal glands)
- Cachexia, cough, dyspnea, hemoptysis, jaundice

Uncommon symptoms
- DIC, paraneoplastic syndromes

HISTORY[4–11]

Age
- Men over the age of 50 are at greatest risk.

Race
- African-American men are at greatest risk.
- Immigration to United States changes disease incidence (from Asian countries, increased incidence correlates with length of residence).

Family History
- First-degree relatives with prostate cancer and age at diagnosis (higher number of relatives and younger age increases risk)
- Familial breast cancer may increase risk.

Other History
- Prior prostate cancer screenings and results of PSA, DRE, biopsies, and other tests performed

Medications
- Assess the patient for use of drugs and herbal or other over-the-counter medications that affect bladder function or reduce PSA (see **Table 4–3**).
- Analgesic use—do a pain assessment.

See **Table 4–2** for information to include in patient history and review of systems.

TABLE 4–2 Information to Include in Patient History and Review of Systems

1. Demographics: age, race, ethnicity, country of origin
2. Family history of prostate cancer; if so, age at diagnosis; other cancers?
3. Prior history of DRE, PSA, prostate biopsies with details of results
4. List current medications (including both prescription, over-the-counter, and herbal medications)
5. Other past and present health problems or illnesses
6. Past history of surgery involving urinary tract; other surgeries
7. History of urinary tract infection(s)
8. History of urinary frequency, urgency, hesitance, incontinence, nocturia, dysuria
9. History of hematuria or hematospermia
10. Any complaints of pain; if so, check location, duration, precipitating and alleviating factors, any associated radiation of pain, focal weakness, numbness, or sphincter disturbances

Source: Roethke SK. Initial assessment and diagnosis. In: Held-Warmkessel, J., ed. *Contemporary Issues in Prostate Cancer: A Nursing Perspective* (2nd ed). Jones and Bartlett Publishers, 2006, 79–106. Reprinted with permission by Jones and Bartlett Publishers.

TABLE 4–3   Drugs That May Cause or Treat Urinary Symptoms

Drug Class	Drug Effects

Anticholinergics
    e.g., Oxybutynin
         Tolterodine
	Relaxes smooth muscle of ureters and bladder walls slowing voiding; used to treat urinary frequency or urge incontinence; could cause urinary retention

Cholinergics e.g., Bethanechol	Increases bladder contractility; used to treat urinary retention

Alpha-adrenergic blockers
    e.g., Terazosin
         Doxazosin
         Tamsulosin
	Improves urinary flow by relaxing prostatic smooth muscle, decreases bladder outlet resistance; used to treat BPH

5-α reductase inhibitors
    e.g., Finasteride
         Dutasteride
	Improves urinary flow and reduces symptoms of BPH; PSA values must be multiplied by 2 to correct for the effect of finasteride

Opioids/Narcotics	Can cause urinary retention
Antiparkinsonism agents	Can cause urinary frequency or retention
Antihistamines	Can cause urinary retention, particularly with preexisting urinary obstruction
Over-the-counter cold/allergy preparations—may contain antihistamines and/or sympathomimetic drugs	Can cause urinary retention, particularly with preexisting urinary obstruction

Source: Roethke SK. Initial assessment and diagnosis. In: Held-Warmkessel, J., ed. *Contemporary Issues in Prostate Cancer: A Nursing Perspective* (2nd ed). Jones and Bartlett Publishers, 2006, 79–106. Reprinted with permission by Jones and Bartlett Publishers.

PHYSICAL EXAMINATION
Digital Rectal Examination (DRE)[12–15]
- Used to determine prostate gland symmetry and texture
- Used with PSA testing to increase sensitivity of disease detection

Procedure
- Position the patient in a side-lying, knee-chest, or bent-over position.
- Assess the anal area.
- Well-lubricated gloved finger is inserted into the rectum.
- Assess rectal sphincter tone.
- Evaluate the rectum for tumors.
- Palpate prostate gland in a clockwise and counterclockwise manner.
- Normal gland is 2.5 cm in length, nontender, and rubbery.
- Cancers are characterized by the presence of abnormal areas—irregularity; stonelike, hard, indurated, flat, or nodular areas; indistinct margins.
- DRE limitation—anterior gland cannot be palpated.
- Small tumors may not be palpable.
- Tumor size often under- or overestimated.

LABORATORY[3, 16–43]

Serum Prostate-Specific Antigen (PSA)

- Reliable test for detection of early prostate cancer
- PSA is specific for prostatic diseases as it is produced only by prostate tissue; benign, malignant, or hyperplastic
- Normal physiologic function produces an enzyme that improves sperm motility.
- PSA half-life in serum $\sim$ 3 days
- PSA normally stays within the prostate gland.
- Causes of increased PSA include prostate cancer, BPH, acute urinary retention, prostatitis, prostate biopsy, and ejaculation (levels higher for longer period of time in older patients).
- PSA levels per gram of prostate cancer tissue are 10x higher than per gram of BPH.

PSA Occurs in Different Molecular Forms

- Bound (complexed) and unbound (free)
- Majority is complexed to antiprotease called α-1-antichymotrypsin, and adequate amounts are present to bind to unbound PSA.
- Uncomplexed PSA is termed free PSA (fPSA).
- Total PSA (tPSA) is composed of a complex form of PSA (cPSA) and a free form of PSA (fPSA).
- Normal level of PSA is 0.0–4.0 ng/mL.
- About 20% of men with prostate cancer have low levels of PSA. DRE and PSA must both be performed to assess for prostate cancer.

Finasteride

- PSA is lowered by finasteride used in the treatment of BPH. Drug interferes with the enzyme 5α-reductase and reduces the conversion of testosterone to dihydrotestosterone (DHT). Because DHT causes prostate growth, reduction of DHT levels results in prostate size reduction. A dose of 5 mg/day is prescribed to reduce symptoms of BPH. As a result of reduced 5α-reductase activity, PSA levels are reduced by approximately 50% with 6 months of drug usage. Finasteride side effects include loss of libido, impotence, breast tenderness, and gynecomastia.

In Men Taking Finasteride

- Double (multiply x 2) the PSA test result, and use the normal PSA range to evaluate for the presence of elevated PSA level and prostate pathology.

Problems with the PSA Test

- PSA levels overlap in patients with prostate cancer and those with nonmalignant prostate diseases.
- PSA results of concern include those between 2 and 10 ng/mL.

Additional PSA Tests Developed to Address PSA Test Problems

PSA density
- Ratio of serum PSA to prostate gland volume
- Determined by TRUS
- Not as reliable as serum PSA results
- May be used as an adjunct in assessing risk
- Measurement of transitional zone density being researched

Age-specific and race-specific PSA reference ranges
- See Chapter 2 for tables for age- and race-specific ranges.
- PSA levels are correlated with age, race, and prostate volume.
- PSA levels are higher in older patients and larger prostate gland volume.
- Use of age-specific reference ranges may improve cancer detection in younger patients.
- Use of race-specific reference ranges may improve cancer detection in African-American patients.

Molecular forms of PSA
fPSA
- Assay developed to determine amount of free (unbound) to total PSA
- Majority of BPH-produced PSA is free.
- Majority of tumor-produced PSA is complexed, and the free level is reduced. The free level is lower and complexed level is higher in men with prostate cancer.
- Results reported as a percentage (ratio of fPSA:tPSA=percent fPSA)
- May be useful in patients with the following: PSA levels 4–10 ng/mL, 10–20 ng/mL, and 2–4 ng/mL, (most useful in 4–40 ng/mL range, reported useful in 2–4 and 10–20 range).
- Use may reduce number of unnecessary biopsies.
- Ongoing research may help determine the most useful % fPSA value and its overall value in patient care.
cPSA
- Level higher in prostate cancer
- Ratios of different PSA molecular forms may be useful adjuncts in patient assessment, but more research is needed.
Pro-PSA[44–49]
- Type of PSA found in transitional and peripheral zones
- Associated with prostate cancer
- May be useful in patients with PSA values of 2–4 ng/mL
- May be useful in diagnosis of aggressive tumors
- More research needed to determine its role and remains investigational
Human glandular kallikrein-2[50–53]
- Serine protease
- Found in prostate tissue
- Breaks PSA molecules
- Level increased in prostate cancer and in poorly differentiated cancers

IMAGING[54]

Purpose
- Identify disease confined to prostate or disease that has spread beyond the gland.
- Assess prostate gland, seminal vesicles, bladder base, rectal wall, and periprostatic tissues.
- Treatment planning

Transrectal Ultrasound
- Performed via rectum
- Use of ultrasound probe and ultrasound energy
- Estimates prostate volume
- Provides prostate needle biopsy guidance

- Guides brachytherapy treatment planning and seed placement at time of implantation

Magnetic Resonance Imaging (MRI) with Endorectal Coil

- Used to determine extent of disease and staging
- Used to evaluate for disease spread to or through the capsule, seminal vesicles, and neurovascular bundle, and regional lymph nodes
- Useful in evaluating patients at risk for extracapsular spread
- Use with spectroscopic imaging under investigation. Spectroscopic imaging identified tissue metabolism of choline and citrate.

Computed Tomography (CT)

- Limited usefulness in low-risk prostate cancer
- More useful in patients with locally advanced disease, Gleason score $\geq$ 8, PSA > 20 ng/mL
- CT used to guide treatment planning for radiation therapy and for CT-guided fine-needle aspiration

Bone Scan[3, 57, 58]

- Used to determine presence of bone metastases
- Recommended for men with PSA $\geq$ 20 ng/mL, Gleason score $\geq$ 8, locally advanced disease or symptomatic disease
- Requires follow-up of suspicious areas by plain radiographs

Positive Emission Tomography[59]

- Currently has no role in evaluation of prostate cancer

BIOPSY[1, 60–76]

- Used to obtain tissue for pathology and staging
- Use of PSA screening identifies tumors that may not be palpable or seen on TRUS; therefore, biopsies need to be taken to identify the areas of disease.
- Sextant pattern of six biopsies are taken in a systematic manner from both sides of the prostate and are performed more often than older core biopsies.

Sextant Biopsies

- Most common approach
- Are performed transrectally in the parasagittal plane
- Are taken from the base, middle, and apex of gland
- Are a minimum of six specimens plus biopsies of hypoechoic areas identified by TRUS
- Are done using an 18-gauge needle on a spring-loaded biopsy gun that makes a loud noise with each activation
- Are TRUS guided
- 20–30% of cancers may be missed, may miss adequate sampling from larger tumors or tumors in the peripheral zone.

Other Biopsy Techniques

- Studied number of specimens obtained and varied from 8 to 23 plus specimens from the lateral aspects of peripheral zone

For patients under age 59, a minimum of 10 biopsies should be obtained plus specimens from the mid lobar apex and base, lateral apex, mid and base.

For patients over age 59, a minimum of eight biopsies are needed and should include the mid lobar apex, lateral base, lateral mid, and lateral apex.
- Biopsy complications such as infection, rectal bleeding, rectal discomfort, hematuria, and vasovagal events are unusual.
- Self-limiting hematuria, hematospermia, hematochezia, and low-grade fever may occur.
- Specimens are sent to pathology for examination and Gleason grading.

Patient Education
- Procedure performed on an outpatient basis
- NSAIDs and ASA are usually stopped 10 days prebiopsy
- Prebiopsy enema, antibiotic (such as a single dose of a long-acting fluoroquinolone)
- Procedure performed in side-lying position
- Under local anesthesia
- DRE followed by ultrasound probe insertion into rectum to guide biopsies
- Patient feels fullness or pressure during procedure; anal probe insertion is the most uncomfortable part of the procedure for many patients.
- Postbiopsy urine specimen may be sent for blood analysis.
- Common side effects are hematuria, hematospermia, and hematochezia.

I thank Sue Roethke, CRNP, for her review of the chapter contents.

References

1. McNeal JE, Redwire EA, Freiha FF, Stamey TA. Zonal distribution of prostatic adenocarcinoma: correlation with histological pattern and directional spread. *Am J Surg Pathol.* 1988;12:897–906.
2. Kim ED, Grahack JT. Clinical symptoms and signs of prostate cancer. In: Vogelzang N, Scardino PT, Shipley WU, Coffey DS, eds. *Genitourinary Oncology.* 2nd ed. Philadelphia, Pa: Lippincott, Williams & Wilkins; 2000:525–532.
3. Ballentine B, Carter HB, Partin AW. Diagnosis and staging of prostate cancer. In: Retik AB, Vaughn ED, Wein AJ, eds. *Campbell's Urology.* 8th ed. Philadelphia, Pa: Saunders; 2002:3055–3079.
4. Parkin DM, Bray F, Ferlay J, Pisano P. Global cancer statistics, 2002. *CA Cancer J Clin.* 2005;55:74–108.
5. Whittemore AF, Wu AH, Kolonel LN, et al. Family history and prostate risk in black, white, and Asian men in the United States and Canada. *Am J Epidemiol.* 1995;141:732–740.
6. Carter BS, Bova GS, Beaty TH, et al. Hereditary prostate cancer: epidemiologic and clinical features. *J Urol.* 1993;150:797–802.
7. Struewing JP, Hartage P, Wacholder S, et al. The risk of cancer associated with specific mutations of BRCA1 and BRCA2 among Ashkenazi Jews. *New Eng J Med.* 1997;336:1401–1408.
8. Liede A, Karkan BY, Narod SA. Cancer risks for male carriers of germline mutations in BRCA1 or BRCA2: a review of the literature. *J Clin Oncol.* 2004;22:735–742.
9. Sinclair CS, Berry D, Scaid D, et al. BRCA1 and BRCA2 have a limited role in familial prostate cancer. *Cancer Res.* 2000;60:1371–1375.
10. Kirchoff T, Kauff ND, Mitra N, et al. BRCA mutations and risk of prostate cancer in Ashkenazi Jews. *Clin Cancer Res.* 2004;10:2918–2921.
11. Parkin DM. Global cancer statistics in the year 2000. *Lancet Oncol.* 2001;2:533–543.

12. Potter SR, Horninger W, Tinzel M, et al. Age, prostate-specific antigen, and digital rectal examination as determinants of the possibility of having prostate cancer. *Urology*. 2001;57:1100–1104.
13. Ellis WJ, Chetner MP, Preston SD, Brawer MK. Diagnosis of prostatic carcinoma: the yield of serum prostate-specific antigen, digital rectal examination and transrectal ultrasonography. *J Urol*. 1994;52:15–20.
14. Bates B, Bickley LS, Hoekelman RA. The anus, rectum, and prostate. *A Guide to Physical Examination and History Taking*. 6th ed. Philadelphia, Pa: Lippincott; 1995:417–425.
15. Brawer MK. The diagnosis of prostate cancer. *Cancer*. 1993;71(suppl):1899–1905.
16. Nadler RB, Humphrey PA, Smith DS, et al. Effect of inflammation and benign prostatic hyperplasia on elevated serum prostate-specific antigen levels. *J Urol*. 1995;154:407–413.
17. Carver BS, Bozeman CB, Williams BJ, Venable DD. The prevalence of men with National Institutes of Health category IV prostatitis and association with serum prostate-specific antigen. *J Urol*. 2003;169:589–591.
18. Benson MC, Whang IS, Pantuck A, et al. Prostate-specific antigen density: a means of distinguishing benign prostatic hypertrophy in prostate cancer. *J Urol*. 1992;147:815–816.
19. Guess HA, Heyse JF, Gormley GJ. The effect of Finasteride on prostate-specific antigen in men with benign prostatic hyperplasia. *Prostate*. 1993;22:31–37.
20. Stenman UH, Alfthan H, and Scandinavian BPH Study Group. Effective long-term treatment with Finasteride on free and total PSA in serum. *J Urol*. 1996;155(Part 2):698a, abstract 1547.
21. Gormley GJ, Ng J, Cook T, et al. Effect of Finasteride on prostate-specific antigen density. *Urology*. 1994;43:53–58.
22. Oesterling JE, Roy J, Agha A, et al. Biologic variability of prostate-specific antigen and its usefulness as a marker for prostate cancer: effects of Finasteride. Finasteride PSA Study Group. *Urology*. 1998;51(4a suppl):58–63.
23. Semjonow A, Roth S, Hamm M, Rather P. Re: non-traumatic elevation of prostate specific antigen following cardiac surgery and extra corporeal cardiopulmonary bypass. *J Urol*. 1995;155:295–296.
24. Deliveliotis C, Alivizatos G, Stavropoulos NJ, et al. Influence of digital examination, cystoscopy, transrectal ultrasonography and needle biopsy on the concentration of prostate-specific antigen. *Urol Int*. 1994;53:186–190.
25. Oesterling JE, Rice DC, Glenski WJ, Bergstralh EJ. Effect of cystoscopy, prostate biopsy and transurethral resection of the prostate on serum prostate-specific antigen concentration. *Urology*. 1993;42:276–280.
26. Tchetgen MB, Song JT, Strawderman M, et al. Ejaculation increases the serum prostate-specific antigen concentration. *Urology*. 1996;47:511–516.
27. Herschman JD, Smith DS, Catalona WJ. Effect of ejaculation on serum total and free prostate-specific antigen concentrations. *Urology*. 1997;50:239–243.
28. Lilja H, Christensson A, Dahlen U, et al. Prostate-specific antigen in serum occurs predominantly in complex with alpha-1-antichymotrypsin. *Clin Chem*. 1991;37:1618–1625.
29. Stenman UH, Leinonen J, Alfthan H, et al. A complex between prostate-specific antigen and a a1-antichymotrypsin is the major form of prostate-specific antigen in serum of patients with prostatic cancer: assay of the complex improves clinical sensitivity for cancer. *Cancer Res*. 1991;51:222–226.

30. Zhang WM, Finne P, Leinonen J, Stenman UH. Characterization and determination of the complex between prostate-specific antigen and alpha-1-protease inhibitor in benign and malignant prostatic diseases. *Scan J Clin Lab Invest.* 2000;(suppl):51–58.

31. Catalona WJ, Hudson PT, Scardino et al. Selection of optimal prostate specific antigen cutoffs for early detection of prostate cancer: receiver operator characteristic curves. *J Urol.* 1994;152:2037–2042.

32. Partin AW, Carter HB, Chan DW, et al. Prostate specific antigen in the staging of localized prostate cancer: influence of tumor differentiation, tumor volume and benign hyperplasia. *J Urol.* 1990;143:747–752.

33. Oesterling JE, Jacobsen SJ, Guess HA, et al. Serum prostate-specific antigen in a community-based population of healthy men: establishment of age-specific reference ranges. *JAMA.* 1993;270:860–864.

34. Partin AW, Criley SR, Subong ENP, et al. Standard versus age-specific prostate specific antigen reference ranges among men with clinically localized prostate cancer: a pathological analysis. *J Urol.* 1996;155:1336–1339.

35. Morgan TO, Jacobsen SJ, McCarthy WF, et al. Age specific reference range for prostate-specific antigen in black men. *New Eng J Med.* 1996;335:304–310.

36. Seaman E, Whang IS, Olsson CA, et al. PSA density (PSAD). Role in patient evaluation and management. *Urol Clinics of North Am.* 1993;20:653–661.

37. Brawer MK, Aramburu EAG, Chen GL, et al. The inability of prostate-specific antigen index to enhance the predictive value of prostate-specific antigen in the diagnosis of prostatic carcinoma. *J Urol.* 1993;150:369–373.

38. Catalona WJ, Richie JP, deKernion JB, et al. Comparison of prostate-specific antigen concentration versus prostate-specific antigen density in the early detection of prostate cancer: receiver operating characteristic curves. *J Urol.* 1994;152:2031–2036.

39. Le Por H, Wang B, Shapiro E. Relationship between prostatic epithelial volume and serum prostate-specific antigen levels. *Urology.* 1994;44:199–205.

40. Catalona WJ, Partin AW, Slawin KM, et al. Use of percentage free prostate-specific antigen to enhance differentiation of prostate cancer from benign disease: a prospective multicenter clinical trial. *JAMA.* 1998;279:1542–1547.

41. Morote J, Trilla E, Esquene S, et al. The percentage free prostate-specific antigen is also useful in men with normal digital rectal examination and serum prostate-specific antigen between 10.1 and 20 ng/ml. *Eur Urol.* 2002;42:333–337.

42. Catalona WJ, Partin AW, Finlay JA, et al. Use of percentage of free prostate-specific antigen to identify men at high risk of prostate cancer when PSA levels are 2.51 to 4.0 ng/ml and digital rectal examination is not suspicious for prostate cancer: an alternative model. *Urology.* 1999;54:220–224.

43. Uzzo RG, Pinover WH, Horwitz EM, et al. Free prostate-specific antigen improves prostate cancer detection in a high-risk population of men with a normal total PSA and digital rectal examination. *Urology.* 2003;61:754–759.

44. Mikolajczyk SD, Marker KM, Millar LS, et al. A truncated precursor form of prostate-specific antigen is a more specific serum marker of prostate cancer. *Cancer Res.* 2001;61:6958–6963.

45. Sokoll LG, Chan DW, Mikolajczyk SD, et al. Proenzyme PSA for the early detection of prostate cancer in the 2.5–4.0 mg/ml total PSA range: preliminary analysis. *J Urol.* 2003;61:274–276.

46. Catalona WJ, Bartsch G, Rittenhouse HG, et al. Serum proPSA improves cancer detection compared to free and complex PSA to men with PSA values from 2–4 ng/ml. *J Urol.* 2003;170:2181–2185.

47. Kahn MA, Partin AW, Rittenhouse HG, et al. Evaluation of proprostate specific antigen for early detection of prostate cancer in men with a total prostate specific antigen range of 4.0-10.0 ng/ml. *J Urol.* 2003;170:723–726.
48. Mikolajczyk SD, Catalona WJ, Evans CL, et al. Proenzyme forms of prostate-specific antigen in serum improved the detection of prostate cancer. *Clin Chem.* 2004;50:1017–1025.
49. Catalona WJ, Bartsch G, Rittenhouse HG, et al. Serum pro-prostate specific antigen preferentially detects aggressive prostate cancers in men with 2-4 ng/ml prostate specific antigen. *J Urol.* 2004;171:2239–2244.
50. Partin AW, Catalona WJ, Finlay JA, et al. Use of the human glandular kallikrein-2 for the detection of prostate cancer: preliminary analysis. *Urology.* 1999;54:839–845.
51. Nam RK, Diamandis EP, Toi A, et al. Serum glandular kallikrein-2 protease levels predict the presence of prostate cancer among men with elevated prostate-specific antigen. *J Crit Oncol.* 2000;18:1036–1042.
52. Darson MF, Pacelli A, Roche P, et al. Human glandular kallikrein-2 (hK2) expression in prostatic intraepithelial neoplasia and adenocarcinoma: a novel prostate cancer marker. *Urology.* 1997;49:857–862.
53. Tremblay RR, Deperthaes D, Tetu B, et al. Immunohistochemical study suggesting a complimentary role of kallikreins hK2 and hK3 (prostate-specific antigen) in the functional analysis of human prostate tumors. *Am J Pathol.* 1997;150:455–459.
54. Adusumilli S, Pretorius ES. Magnetic resonance imaging of prostate cancer. *Seminars Urol Oncol.* 2002;20:192–210.
55. Yu KK, Scheidler J, Hricak H, et al. Prostate cancer: prediction of extracapsular extension with endorectal MR imaging and 3-dimensional proton MR spectroscopic imaging. *Radiol.* 1999;213:481–488.
56. Kurhanewicz J, Vigneron DB, Males RG, et al. The prostate: MR imaging and spectroscopy. Present and future. *Radiol Clin North Am.* 2000;38:115–138.
57. Abuzallouf S, Dayes I, Lukka H. Baseline staging of newly diagnosed prostate cancer: a summary of the literature. *J Urol.* 2004;171:2122–2124.
58. Albertsen PC, Hanley JA, Harlen LC, et al. The positive yield of imaging studies in the evaluation of men with newly diagnosed prostate cancer: a population based analysis. *J Urol.* 2000;163:1138–1143.
59. Shvarts O, Han KR, Seltzer M, et al. Positive emission tomography in urologic oncology. *Cancer Control.* 2002;9:335–342.
60. Hodge KK, McNeal JE, Terris MK, et al. Random systematic versus directed ultrasound-guided transrectal core biopsies of the prostate. *J Urol.* 1989;142:71–75.
61. Uzzo RG, Wei JT, Waldbaum RS, et al. The influence of prostate size on cancer detection. *Urology.* 1995;46:831–836.
62. Eskew LA, Bare RL, McCullough DL. Systematic 5 region prostate biopsy is superior to sextant method for diagnosing carcinoma of the prostate. *J Urol.* 1997;156:199–202.
63. Stewart CS, Leibovich BC, Weaver AL, Lieber MM. Prostate cancer diagnosis using a saturation needle biopsy technique after previous negative sextant biopsies. *J Urol.* 2001;166:86–91.
64. Levine MA, Ittman M, Melamed J, Lepor H. Two consecutive sets of transrectal ultrasound guided sextant biopsies of the prostate for detection of prostate cancer. *J Urol.* 1998;159:471–475.
65. Babaian RJ, Toi A, Kamoi K, et al. A comparative analysis of sextant and and extended 11-core multisite directed biopsy strategy. *J Urol.* 2000;163:152–157.

66. Presti JC Jr, Chang JJ, Bhargava V, Shinohara K. The optimal systematic prostate biopsy scheme should include 8 rather than 6 biopsies: results of a perspective clinical trial. *J Urol.* 2000;163:163–166.
67. Naughton CK, Miller DC, Mager DE, Ornstein DK, Catalano WJ. A prospective randomized trial comparing 6 versus 12 biopsy cores: impact on cancer detection. *J Urol.* 2000;164:388–392.
68. Eskew LA, Woodruff RD, Bare RL, McCullough DL. Prostate cancer diagnosed by the five region biopsy method is significant disease. *J Urol.* 1998;160:794–796.
69. Chan TY, Chan DY, Lecksell K, Stutzman RE, Epstein JI. Does increased needle biopsy sampling of the prostate detect a higher number of potentially insignificant tumors? *J Urol.* 2001;166:2181–2184.
70. Presti JC Jr, O'Dowd GJ, Miller M, et al. Extended peripheral zone biopsy schemes increase cancer detection rates and minimize variance in prostate-specific antigen and age-related cancer rates: results of a community multi-practice study. *J Urol.* 2003;169:125–129.
71. Lindert KA, Kabalin JN, Terris MK. Bacteremia and bacteriuria after transrectal ultrasound guided prostate biopsy. *J Urol.* 2000;164:76–80.
72. Carey JM, Korman HJ. Transrectal ultrasound guided biopsy of the prostate. Do enemas decrease clinically significant complications? *J Urol.* 2001;166:82–85.
73. Shandera KC, Thibault GP, Deshon GE Jr. Efficacy of one dose fluoroquinolone before prostate biopsy. *Urology.* 1998;52:641–646.
74. Oliffe J. Transrectal prostate biopsy (TRUS-Bx): patient perspectives. *Uro Nurs.* 2004;24:395–400.
75. Rodriguez LV, Terris MK. Risks and complications of transrectal ultrasound guided needle biopsy: a prospective study and review of the literature. *J Urol.* 1998;160:2115–2120.
76. Herget EJ, Salliken JC, Donnelly BJ, et al. Transrectal ultrasound-guided biopsy of the prostate: relation between ASA use and bleeding complications. *Can Assoc Radiol J.* 1999;50:173–176.

Chapter 5
Staging

INTRODUCTION
Purposes of Staging[1]
- Describe extent of disease
- Guide therapy
- Extent of disease in newly diagnosed patients correlates with prognosis.

Pretreatment staging includes
- PSA
- DRE
- Histologic grade
- Imaging studies
- Use of nomograms

CLASSIFICATION SYSTEMS
Whitmore-Jewett System[2-6]
- Commonly used in North America
- Four stages, A through D
- Has been revised but limitations remain
- Easy to use
- Provides prognostic information for clinically localized disease
- See **Table 5–1.**

Tumor Node Metastasis (TNM) Staging System
- Commonly used outside North America
- More difficult to use

1992 American Joint Committee on Cancer/International Union Against Cancer (AJCC/UICC) TNM System[6-9]
- See **Table 5–1.**
- T1c tumors are identified by elevated prostate-specific antigen (PSA) and transrectal ultrasound (TRUS).
- Similar to T2 lesions in terms of clinical importance

Developed to
- Be used in daily medical practice
- Be flexible
- Keep the basic principles of the Whitmore system

Limitations of the AJCC/UICC TNM System[6, 8, 10]
- Use of TRUS for staging
- Needs to be revised when new tests become available
- Understaging common

Table 5–1   Comparison of TNM and Whitmore-Jewett Staging Systems

TNM	Description	Whitmore-Jewett	Description
TX	Primary tumor cannot be assessed	None*	None
T0	No evidence of primary tumor	None	None
T1	Clinically unapparent tumor—not palpable or visible by imaging	A	Same as TNM
T1a	Tumor found incidentally in tissue removed at TUR; 5% or less of tissue is cancerous	A1	Same as TNM
T1b	Tumor found incidentally at TUR; more than 5% of tissue is cancerous	A2	Same as TNM
T1c	Tumor identified by prostate needle biopsy because of PSA elevation	None	None
T2	Palpable tumor confined within the prostate	B	Same as TNM
T2a	Tumor involves half a lobe or less	B1N	Tumor involves half of a lobe or less; surrounded by normal tissue
T2b	Tumor involves more than half a lobe but not both lobes	B1	Tumor involves less than one lobe
T2c	Tumor involves both lobes	B2	Tumor involves one entire lobe or more
T3	Palpable tumor extending through prostate capsule and/or involving seminal vesicle(s)	C1	Tumor < 6 cm in diameter
T3a	Unilateral extracapsular extension	C1	Same as TNM
T3b	Bilateral extracapsular extension	C1	Same as TNM
T3c	Tumor invades seminal vesicle(s)	C1	Same as TNM
T4	Tumor is fixed or invades adjacent structures other than seminal vesicles	C2	Tumor > 6 cm in diameter
T4a	Tumor invades bladder neck and/or external sphincter and/or rectum	C2	Same as TNM
T4b	Tumor invades levator muscles and/or is fixed to pelvic wall	C2	Same as TNM
N	Involvement of regional lymph nodes	D1	Same as TNM
None	None	D0	Elevation of prostatic acid phosphatase only (enzymatic assay)

continues

Table 5–1 Comparison of TNM and Whitmore-Jewett Staging Systems, continued

TNM	Description	Whitmore-Jewett	Description
NX	Regional lymph nodes cannot be assessed	None	None
N0	No regional lymph node metastases	None	None
N1	Metastasis in a single regional lymph node, < 2 cm in greatest dimension	D1	Same as TNM
N2	Metastasis in a single regional lymph node, > 2 cm but not > 5 cm in greatest dimension, or multiple regional lymph nodes, none > 5 cm in greatest dimension	D1	Same as TNM
N3	Metastasis in a regional lymph node > 5 cm in greatest dimension	D1	Same as TNM
M	Distant metastatic spread	D2	Same as TNM
MX	Presence of distant metastases cannot be assessed	None	None
M0	No distant metastases	None	None
M1	Distant metastases	D2	Same as TNM
M1a	Involvement of nonregional lymph nodes	D2	Same as TNM
M1b	Involvement of bones	D2	Same as TNM
M1c	Involvement of other distant sites	D2	Same as TNM
None	None	D3	Hormone refractory disease

None, no comparable category; TUR, transurethral resection; PSA, prostate-specific antigen.
Source: Adapted from Ballentine-Carter H, Carter AW. Prostate cancer staging. In: Walsh PC, Retik AB, Vaughn ED, Wein AJ, eds. *Campbell's Urology.* 8th ed. Philadelphia: WB Saunders, 2002, p. 3065. Reprinted with permission from Elsevier.

Benefits of the AJCC/UICC TNM System[4, 11]

- Accurate and practical
- Large number of tumor classifications

CLINICAL STAGING[12, 13]

Tumor (T) is assessed by digital rectal examination, tumor markers, pathology, diagnostic imaging, and pelvic lymphadenectomy.

Digital Rectal Examination (DRE)[1, 13]

- Easy assessment to perform
- Operator dependent
- Subjective examination
- Used in clinical staging of tumor despite its lack of specificity and sensitivity in determining the presence of disease and its extent

Serum Tumor Markers[6, 14]

Prostatic acid phosphatase (PAP)
- Adds little to clinical staging
- Correlated with disease stage
- Elevated in presence of extracapsular disease, metastatic disease, after DRE, and in prostatitis
- Rarely increased in presence of organ-confined disease
- In patients with elevated PAP but normal bone scan, negative lymph nodes, and localized disease, progression can be predicted within the next 18 months.
- Increased in 67% of patients with disease outside the prostate capsule

Prostate-specific antigen (PSA)[15–17]
- Amount of PSA produced by prostate cells varies.
- Amount of PSA produced per gram of prostate tissue is higher in malignant disease (3.5 ng/mL/g) than in benign disease (0.3 ng/mL/g).
- High-grade, high-volume cancers may make less PSA.
- PSA levels are often higher with advanced stages of disease.
- If PSA is < 4.0 ng/mL, cancer is usually confined to the prostate.
- If PSA is > 10 ng/mL, capsular penetration is present in > 50% of patients.
- If PSA is > 50 ng/mL, cancer has spread to the lymph nodes in a majority of men.
- Poorly differentiated cancer cells may not manufacture PSA.
- Using PSA alone to accurately predict stage is not possible.

Transrectal Ultrasonography (TRUS)[8, 9, 18]

- Used to guide biopsies of the prostate
- Use in staging cancer limited by difficulty in separating benign from malignant tumors, understaging of tumors, and operator dependency

Bone Scan[13, 19]

- Frequently used in staging disease
- Provides baseline assessment of bones
- In men with no bone pain and a PSA level > 10 ng/mL, bone scan will be positive infrequently.

Computed Tomography[13, 20]

- Not as good as DRE and TRUS for staging
- May be done with fine-needle aspiration (FNA)
- May be useful in evaluating men with abnormal DRE, PSA > 25ng/mL, and a high-grade tumor or lymph node > 6 mm.

Magnetic Resonance Imaging (MRI)[8]

- Provides information on pelvic lymph nodes
- Use with endorectal coil improves ability to detect lymph node and seminal vesicle spread.

Pelvic Lymphadenectomy[21, 22]

- May be done by laparoscope or at time of radical prostatectomy to accurately stage lymph nodes
- Not indicated in patients with a PSA < 5 ng/mL; Gleason score < 5; or PSA 25 ng/mL, Gleason score of 7 with negative DRE
- Indicated in patients with enlarged lymph nodes on diagnostic imaging; PSA > 20 ng/mL; Gleason score 8–10; or T3 or T4 disease

SIGNIFICANCE OF TUMOR STAGING[23]

- Men with disease limited to the prostate have better survival than men with disease that has spread beyond the gland.
- Pathologic assessment of tumor volume, grade, and size is needed to distinguish between clinically significant cancers and incidental cancers.
- Determining which men with early stage prostate cancer to treat cannot be accurately predicted by clinical data
- It is difficult to determine which tumors will behave in a benign manner compared to those that will behave aggressively and require treatment.
- Serum PSA, Gleason score, and T stage are currently the best predictors of outcome.
- More research is needed to accurately predict tumor behavior.
- Efforts need to be made to differentiate tumors with benign behavior that do not require aggressive therapy from those that require treatment.

PATHOLOGIC STAGE[2, 12, 13]

- No up-to-date pathologic staging system is available for prostate cancer.
- Pathologic staging of tumor requires documentation of extent of disease from surgical specimens—prostate gland and seminal vesicles
- Extent of spread to surrounding tissues is reported.
- Pathologic staging of node (N) requires documentation of extent of disease from pelvic lymph nodes.

HISTOLOGIC GRADE[2, 4, 9, 13, 24, 25]

- Aids in predicting pathologic grade and prognosis
- Based on microscopic examination of tissue specimens and the glandular pattern
- Gleason system of five grades, grades 1 to 5
- Grade 1 tumors are well differentiated
- Grade 5 tumors are poorly differentiated
- Each tumor is given two grades, one for each of the two most dominant cellular patterns in the specimen. These two numbers are added together to give a total Gleason score or sum of 2–10 (see **Table 5–2**).

TABLE 5–2 Histologic Grade

Grade (G)	Description
GX	Grade cannot be assessed
G1c	Well differentiated (slight anaplasia) (Gleason 2–4)
G2	Moderately differentiated (moderate anaplasia) (Gleason 5–6)
G3–4	Poorly differentiated or undifferentiated (marked anaplasia) (Gleason 7–10)

If grouping of Gleason scores is necessary for research purposes, the following grouping is suggested: Gleason score 2–4, well differentiated; 5–6, moderately differentiated; 7, moderately poorly differentiated; 8–10, poorly differentiated.

Source: Adapted with permission of the American Joint Committee on Cancer (AJCC), Chicago, Ill. The original source for this material is the *AJCC Cancer Staging Manual*, 6th edition (2002) published by Lippincott-Raven Publishers, Philadelphia, Pa.

TABLE 5-3 Clinical Stage T1c (nonpalpable, PSA elevated)

PSA Range (ng/mL)	Pathologic Stage	Gleason Score				
		2–4	5–6	3 + 4 = 7	4 + 3 = 7	8–10
0–2.5	Organ confined	95 (89–99)	90 (88–93)	79 (74–85)	71 (62–79)	66 (54–76)
	Extraprostatic extension	5 (1–11)	9 (7–12)	17 (13–23)	25 (18–34)	28 (20–38)
	Seminal vesicle (+)	—	0 (0–1)	2 (1–5)	2 (1–5)	4 (1–10)
	Lymph node (+)	—	—	1 (0–2)	1 (0–4)	1 (0–4)
2.6–4.0	Organ confined	92 (82–98)	84 (81–86)	68 (62–74)	58 (48–67)	52 (41–63)
	Extraprostatic extension	8 (2–18)	15 (13–18)	27 (22–33)	37 (29–46)	40 (31–50)
	Seminal vesicle (+)	—	1 (0–1)	4 (2–7)	4 (1–7)	6 (3–12)
	Lymph node (+)	—	—	1 (0–2)	1 (0–3)	1 (0–4)
4.1–6.0	Organ confined	90 (78–98)	80 (78–83)	63 (58–68)	52 (43–60)	46 (36–56)
	Extraprostatic extension	10 (2–22)	19 (16–21)	32 (27–36)	42 (35–50)	45 (36–54)
	Seminal vesicle (+)	—	1 (0–1)	3 (2–5)	3 (1–6)	5 (3–9)
	Lymph node (+)	—	0 (0–1)	2 (1–3)	3 (1–6)	3 (1–6)
6.1–10.0	Organ confined	87 (73–97)	75 (72–77)	54 (49–59)	43 (35–51)	37 (28–36)
	Extraprostatic extension	13 (3–27)	23 (21–25)	36 (32–40)	47 (40–54)	48 (39–57)
	Seminal vesicle (+)	—	2 (2–3)	8 (6–11)	8 (4–12)	13 (8–19)
	Lymph node (+)	—	0 (0–1)	2 (1–3)	2 (1–4)	3 (1–5)
>10.0	Organ confined	80 (61–95)	62 (58–64)	37 (32–42)	27 (21–34)	22 (16–30)
	Extraprostatic extension	20 (5–39)	33 (30–36)	43 (38–48)	51 (44–59)	50 (42–59)
	Seminal vesicle (+)	—	4 (3–5)	12 (9–17)	11 (6–17)	17 (10–25)
	Lymph node (+)	—	2 (1–3)	8 (5–11)	10 (5–17)	11 (5–18)

PSA, prostate-specific antigen.

Numbers represent probability (%). Dash represents lack of sufficient data to calculate probability.

Source: Partin AW, Mangold LA, Lamm DM, et al. Contemporary update of prostate cancer staging nomograms (Partin tables) for the new millennium. *Urology.* 2001; 58:843–848.

TABLE 5–4 Clinical Stage T2a (palpable < ½ of one lobe)

PSA Range (ng/mL)	Pathologic Stage	Gleason Score					
		2–4	5–6	3 + 4 = 7	4 + 3 = 7	8–10
0–2.5	Organ confined	91 (79–98)	81 (77–85)	64 (56–71)	53 (43–63)	47 (35–59)
	Extraprostatic extension	9 (2–21)	17 (13–21)	29 (23–36)	40 (30–49)	42 (32–53)
	Seminal vesicle (+)	—	1 (0–2)	5 (1–9)	4 (1–9)	7 (2–16)
	Lymph node (+)	—	0 (0–1)	2 (0–5)	3 (0–8)	3 (0–9)
2.6–4.0	Organ confined	85 (69–96)	71 (66–75)	50 (43–57)	39 (30–48)	33 (24–44)
	Extraprostatic extension	15 (4–31)	27 (23–31)	41 (35–48)	52 (43–61)	53 (44–63)
	Seminal vesicle (+)	—	2 (1–3)	7 (3–12)	6 (2–12)	10 (4–18)
	Lymph node (+)	—	0 (0–1)	2 (0–4)	2 (0–6)	3 (0–8)
4.1–6.0	Organ confined	81 (63–95)	66 (62–70)	44 (39–50)	33 (25–41)	28 (20–37)
	Extraprostatic extension	19 (5–37)	32 (28–36)	46 (40–52)	56 (48–64)	58 (49–66)
	Seminal vesicle (+)	—	1 (1–2)	5 (3–8)	5 (2–8)	8 (4–13)
	Lymph node (+)	—	1 (0–2)	4 (2–7)	6 (3–11)	6 (2–12)
6.1–10.0	Organ confined	76 (56–94)	58 (54–61)	35 (30–40)	25 (19–32)	21 (15–28)
	Extraprostatic extension	24 (6–44)	37 (34–41)	49 (43–54)	58 (51–66)	57 (48–65)
	Seminal vesicle (+)	—	4 (3–5)	13 (9–18)	11 (6–17)	17 (11–26)
	Lymph node (+)	—	1 (0–2)	3 (2–6)	5 (2–8)	5 (2–10)
>10.0	Organ confined	65 (43–89)	42 (38–46)	20 (17–24)	14 (10–18)	11 (7–15)
	Extraprostatic extension	35 (11–57)	47 (43–52)	49 (43–55)	55 (46–64)	52 (41–62)
	Seminal vesicle (+)	—	6 (4–8)	16 (11–22)	13 (7–20)	19 (12–29)
	Lymph node (+)	—	4 (3–7)	14 (9–21)	18 (10–27)	17 (9–29)

PSA, prostate-specific antigen.
Numbers represent probability (%). Dash represents lack of sufficient data to calculate probability.
Source: Partin AW, Mangold LA, Lamm DM, et al. Contemporary update of prostate cancer staging nomograms (Partin tables) for the new millennium. *Urology.* 2001; 58:843–848.

TABLE 5-5 Clinical Stage T2b (palpable > $1/2$ of one lobe, not on both lobes)

PSA Range (ng/mL)	Pathologic Stage	Gleason Score				
		2-4	5-6	3 + 4 = 7	4 + 3 = 7	8-10
0-2.5	Organ confined	88 (73-97)	75 (69-81)	54 (46-63)	43 (33-54)	37 (26-49)
	Extraprostatic extension	12 (3-27)	22 (17-28)	35 (28-43)	45 (35-56)	46 (35-58)
	Seminal vesicle (+)	—	2 (0-3)	6 (2-12)	5 (1-11)	9 (2-20)
	Lymph node (+)	—	1 (0-2)	4 (0-10)	6 (0-14)	6 (0-16)
2.6-4.0	Organ confined	80 (61-95)	63 (57-69)	41 (33-48)	30 (22-39)	25 (17-34)
	Extraprostatic extension	20 (5-39)	34 (28-40)	47 (40-55)	57 (47-67)	57 (46-68)
	Seminal vesicle (+)	—	2 (1-4)	9 (4-15)	7 (3-14)	12 (5-22)
	Lymph node (+)	—	1 (0-2)	3 (0-8)	4 (0-12)	5 (0-14)
4.1-6.0	Organ confined	75 (55-93)	57 (52-63)	35 (29-40)	25 (18-32)	21 (14-29)
	Extraprostatic extension	25 (7-45)	39 (33-44)	51 (44-57)	60 (50-68)	59 (49-69)
	Seminal vesicle (+)	—	2 (1-3)	7 (4-11)	5 (3-9)	9 (4-16)
	Lymph node (+)	—	2 (1-3)	7 (4-13)	10 (5-18)	10 (4-20)
6.1-10.0	Organ confined	69 (47-91)	49 (43-54)	26 (22-31)	19 (14-25)	15 (10-21)
	Extraprostatic extension	31 (9-53)	44 (39-49)	52 (46-58)	60 (52-68)	57 (48-67)
	Seminal vesicle (+)	—	5 (3-8)	16 (10-22)	13 (7-20)	19 (11-29)
	Lymph node (+)	—	2 (1-3)	6 (4-10)	8 (5-14)	8 (4-16)
> 10.0	Organ confined	57 (35-86)	33 (28-38)	14 (11-17)	9 (6-13)	7 (4-10)
	Extraprostatic extension	43 (14-65)	52 (46-56)	47 (40-53)	50 (40-60)	46 (36-59)
	Seminal vesicle (+)	—	8 (5-11)	17 (12-24)	13 (8-21)	19 (12-29)
	Lymph node (+)	—	8 (5-12)	22 (15-30)	27 (16-39)	27 (14-40)

PSA, prostate-specific antigen.

Numbers represent probability (%). Dash represents lack of sufficient data to calculate probability.

Source: Partin AW, Mangold LA, Lamm DM, et al. Contemporary update of prostate cancer staging nomograms (Partin tables) for the new millennium. Urology. 2001, 58:843–848.

TABLE 5-6 Clinical Stage T2c (palpable on both lobes)

PSA Range (ng/mL)	Pathologic Stage	Gleason Score				
		2-4	5-6	3 + 4 = 7	4 + 3 = 7	8-10
0-2.5	Organ confined	86 (71-97)	73 (63-81)	51 (38-63)	39 (26-54)	34 (21-48)
	Extraprostatic extension	14 (3-29)	24 (17-33)	36 (26-48)	45 (32-59)	47 (33-61)
	Seminal vesicle (+)	—	1 (0-4)	5 (1-13)	5 (1-12)	8 (2-19)
	Lymph node (+)	—	1 (0-4)	6 (0-18)	9 (0-26)	10 (0-27)
2.6-4.0	Organ confined	78 (58-94)	61 (50-70)	38 (27-50)	27 (18-40)	23 (14-34)
	Extraprostatic extension	22 (6-42)	36 (27-45)	48 (37-59)	57 (44-70)	57 (44-70)
	Seminal vesicle (+)	—	2 (1-5)	8 (2-17)	6 (2-16)	10 (3-22)
	Lymph node (+)	—	1 (0-4)	5 (0-15)	7 (0-21)	8 (0-22)
4.1-6.0	Organ confined	73 (52-93)	55 (44-64)	31 (23-41)	21 (14-31)	18 (11-28)
	Extraprostatic extension	27 (7-48)	40 (32-50)	50 (40-60)	57 (43-68)	57 (43-70)
	Seminal vesicle (+)	—	2 (1-4)	13 (6-23)	11 (4-21)	16 (6-29)
	Lymph node (+)	—	3 (1-7)	12 (5-23)	16 (6-32)	16 (6-33)
6.1-10.0	Organ confined	67 (45-91)	46 (36-56)	24 (17-32)	16 (10-24)	13 (8-20)
	Extraprostatic extension	33 (9-55)	36 (37-55)	52 (42-61)	58 (46-69)	56 (43-69)
	Seminal vesicle (+)	—	5 (2-9)	13 (6-23)	11 (4-21)	16 (6-29)
	Lymph node (+)	—	3 (1-6)	10 (5-18)	13 (6-25)	13 (5-26)
>10.0	Organ confined	54 (32-85)	30 (21-38)	11 (7-17)	7 (4-12)	6 (3-10)
	Extraprostatic extension	46 (15-68)	51 (42-60)	42 (30-55)	43 (29-59)	41 (27-57)
	Seminal vesicle (+)	—	6 (2-12)	13 (6-24)	10 (3-20)	15 (5-28)
	Lymph node (+)	—	13 (6-22)	33 (18-49)	38 (20-58)	38 (20-59)

PSA, prostate-specific antigen.

Numbers represent probability (%). Dash represents lack of sufficient data to calculate probability.

Source: Partin AW, Mangold LA, Lamm DM, et al. Contemporary update of prostate cancer staging nomograms (Partin tables) for the new millennium. Urology. 2001; 58:843-848.

- The most common or primary grade is a significant factor used to place patients in prognostic groups.
- Patients with a score of 4 + 3 typically have a worse prognosis than patients with a score of 3 + 4 even though both total 7.
- Tumors with lower Gleason scores (2–4) are more likely to be organ-confined than higher Gleason score (7–10) tumors.
- Gleason scores of 2–4 and 8–10 correlate with final pathology, but those scores in between do not.

COMBINING CLINICAL FACTORS TO PREDICT PATHOLOGICAL STAGE5

- Clinical stage, Gleason score, and serum PSA predict final pathologic stage. Tables and nomograms have been developed and update and aid in determining probability of final pathologic stage. These can be useful tools when educating patients with a new prostate cancer diagnosis about treatment options and outcomes (see **Tables 5–3** through **5–6**).

References

1. Hernandez J, Thompson IM. Diagnosis and treatment of prostate cancer. *Medical Clinics of North America.* 2004; 88:267–279.
2. Carter HB, Partin AW. Diagnosing and staging of prostate cancer. In: Walsh PC, Retik AB, Stamey TA, et al., eds. *Campbell's Urology.* 8th ed. Philadelphia, Pa: WB Saunders; 2002:3055–3079.
3. Levy D, Resnick M. Staging of prostate cancer. In: Raghavan D, Scher H, Leibel SA, Lange PH, eds. *Principle and Practices of Genitourinary Oncology.* Philadelphia, Pa: Lippincott-Raven; 1997:473–490.
4. Zagars GK, Geara FB, Pollack A, von Eschenbach AC. The T classification of clinically localized prostate cancer. *Cancer.* 1994;73:1904–1912.
5. Jewett H. The present status of radical prostatectomy for stages A and B prostate cancer. *Urol Clin North Am.* 1975;5:108–122.
6. Graham SD. Critical assessment of prostate cancer staging. *Cancer.* 1992;70: 269–274.
7. Ohori M, Wheeler T, Scardino P. The New American Joint Committee on Cancer and International Union Against Cancer TNM classification of prostate cancer. *Cancer.* 1994;74:104–114.
8. Kozlowski J M. Carcinoma of the prostate. In: Gillenwater JY, Grayhack J, Howards SS, Mitchell ME, eds. *Adult and Pediatric Urology.* Philadelphia, Pa: Lippincott Williams & Wilkins; 2002:1471–1655.
9. Kozlowski J, Grayhack J. Carcinoma of the prostate. In: Gillenwater J, Grayhack J, Howards SS, Duckett J, eds. *Adult Urology.* St. Louis, Mo: CV Mosby; 1996: 1575–1692.
10. Bostwick D, Amin M. Male reproductive system: Prostate and seminal vesicle. In: Damjanov I, Linder J, eds. *Anderson's Pathology.* St. Louis, Mo: CV Mosby; 1996:2197–2230.
11. McLeod DG. Prostate cancer: Past, present and future. In: Dawson N, Vogelzang N, eds. *Prostate Cancer.* New York. Wiley-Liss; 1994:1–18.
12. Fleming J, Cooper J, Henson D, et al, eds. *Prostate: AJCC Cancer Staging Handbook.* 5th ed. Philadelphia, Pa: Lippincott-Raven; 1998:204–211.
13. O'Dowd G, Veltri R, Orozco R, et al. Update on the appropriate staging evaluation for newly diagnosed prostate cancer. *J Urol.* 1997;158:687–698.

14. Canto EL, Shariat SF, Slawin KM. Biochemical staging of prostate cancer. *Urol Clin North Am.* 2003;30:263–277.
15. Partin A, Yoo J, Carter HB, et al. The use of PSA clinical stage and Gleason score to predict pathologic stage in men with localized prostate cancer. *J Urol.* 1993;150: 110–114.
16. Partin AW, Oesterling J. The clinical usefulness of PSA: Update 1994. *J Urol.* 1994;152:1358–1368.
17. Partin AW, Carter HB, Chan DW, et al. Prostate-specific antigen in the staging of localized prostate cancer: Influence of tumor differentiation, tumor volume and benign hyperplasia. *J Urol.* 1990;143:747–752.
18. Brawer M, Chetner M. Ultrasonography of the prostate and biopsy. In: Walsh PC, Vaughn ED Jr, Wein A, eds. *Campbell's Urology.* 7th ed. Philadelphia, Pa: WB Saunders; 1998:2506–2517.
19. Oesterling J, Martin S, Bergstralh E, Lowe F. The use of prostate-specific antigen in staging patients with newly diagnosed prostate cancer. *JAMA.* 1993;269:57–60.
20. Rees M, Resnick M, Oesterling J. Use of prostate-specific antigen, Gleason score and digital rectal examination in staging patients with newly diagnosed prostate cancer. *Urol Clin North Am.* 1997;24:379–386.
21. Montie J, Meyers S. Defining the ideal tumor marker for prostate cancer. *Urol Clin North Am.* 1997;24:247–259.
22. Miller DC, Hafez KS, Stewart A, et al. Prostate carcinoma presentation, diagnosis and staging. *Cancer.* 2003; 98:1169–1177.
23. Corless CL. Evaluating early-stage prostate cancer. *Hematol Oncol Clin North Am.* 1996;10:565–579.
24. Epstein J. Pathology of adenocarcinoma of the prostate. In: Walsh PC, Retik AB, Vaughn ED, Wein A, eds. *Campbell's Urology.* 7th ed. Philadelphia, Pa: WB Saunders; 1998:2497–2505.
25. Presti JC. Neoplasms of the prostate gland. In: Tanagho EA, McAninck JA, eds. *Smith's General Urology.* 6th ed. New York. Lange Medical Books, McGraw-Hill; 2004:367–385.
26. Partin AW, Mangold LA, Lamm DM, et al. Contemporary update of prostate cancer-staging nomograms (Partin tables) for the new millennium. *Urology.* 2001;58: 843–848.

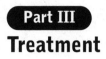

Treatment

Treatment Decision Making

INTRODUCTION

Many patients have more than one treatment option. A wide variety of factors are taken into consideration when making treatment recommendations and the final decision about prostate cancer treatment.

Factors Include

- Treatment efficacy for a given patient
- Risk of complications for a given patient
- Patient preference
- Patient concern about complication profile of a given treatment option such as impotency, incontinence, bowel injury, and change in self-esteem
- Risk of surgical and anesthesia complications
- Patient age
- Expected survival
- Coexisting medical diagnoses
- Method of diagnosis (screening versus presence of symptoms)
- Stage
- Tumor factors
- Expected side effects

PATIENT DATA COLLECTION

- Age
- Disease of older men
- Median age at diagnosis is 72 years.
- Patients may die of other medical causes prior to experiencing problems with their prostate cancer.
- Patient age and expected survival prior to the cancer diagnosis should be considered when making treatment decisions.

Coexisting Medical Problems[1-3]

- Aggressive treatment of prostate cancer is appropriate for men < 70 years of age who have no comorbid medical factors. Comorbid medical factors include cardiac, pulmonary, renal, or cerebrovascular disease. Men with these comorbid factors are more likely to succumb to the medical problem than to prostate cancer. On the other hand, younger men (< 70 years of age) without comorbidities are more likely to benefit from therapy.

Patients Screened by Prostate-Specific Antigen[4-6]

- Prostate cancer identified in asymptomatic men because screening prostate-specific antigen (PSA) tests are staged T1c.

An unresolved issue is whether PSA screening for nonpalpable cancers improves long-term survival. PSA screening reveals cancers that have a lower PSA, lower stage, and lower grade. Currently, it is not known whether a clinically significant cancer would evolve if the cancer is left untreated. More research is needed to clarify this concern.

Stage[7–9]

- Predicts survival
- Organ-confined disease has > 5-year median survival.
- Locally advanced disease has about a 5-year median survival.
- Metastatic cancer has a 1- to 3-year median survival.
- Lymph node metastases carry a poorer prognosis, and thus lymphadenectomy should be considered prior to definitive surgical procedures.
- Seminal vesical disease predicts lymph node metastasis, and a biopsy of the seminal vesicles may be appropriate.
- Gleason score and serum prostatic acid phosphatase predict capsular penetration, seminal vesical involvement, and regional nodal metastases in patients with clinically localized disease.

Tumor Factors[10–12]

- Tumor differentiation and histologic growth pattern correlate with survival and risk of metastases.
- Gleason score is useful in treatment decision making.
- Low Gleason score tumors are less likely to metastasize.
- High Gleason score tumors are more likely to metastasize and recur.
- Low Gleason score tumors are less likely to have an impact on survival.
- High Gleason score tumors are more likely to have an impact on survival.
- Tetraploid and aneuploid tumors have a worse outcome than diploid tumors.

Tumor Markers[13, 14]

- PSA is very useful marker for prostate cancer. It is used to assess prognosis and in monitoring men after treatment, as rising PSA levels predict disease recurrence.
- Elevated serum acid phosphatase is a poor prognostic indicator.

TREATMENT OPTIONS

For many men with localized disease, treatment results in long disease-free survival, but some men develop metastatic disease. For men with locally advanced and metastatic disease, treatment is both beneficial and palliative.

Watchful Waiting[15, 16]

Candidates include men with
- Advanced age and no symptoms
- Comorbid medical problems and low-grade and early stage tumors
- Cancer found at time of surgery for presumed benign prostatic disease
- Well- or moderately-well differentiated tumors localized to the prostate
- Low-grade tumors

SURGERY

Radical Prostatectomy

Candidates include men
- Under age 70
- In good medical health
- Without metastatic disease
- Wanting surgical intervention

- Approaches include retropubic or perineal, preceded by lymph node dissection. If nodes contain metastatic disease, prostatectomy may not be performed.

Pathologic staging of resected specimen
- If disease is confined to the prostate gland, recurrence is unusual.
- Recurrence rates are higher in men with extracapsular disease or positive specimen margins. These patients may be offered postoperative radiation therapy or hormonal manipulation. The impact of additional therapy is unclear.

Laparoscopic Radical Prostatectomy

- Could be an alternative to traditional prostatectomy, but longer follow-up is needed.[17]

Cryosurgery

- Candidates include patients with other medical problems. Role as cancer treatment is not well defined.
- May cause serious complications

External Beam Radiation Therapy[18–22]

Candidates include patients with
- Prostate cancer stages I, II, or III; organ confined or confined to surrounding tissues
- Negative bone scan
- May have undergone staging of lymph nodes by laparoscopy or by CT scan-directed needle biopsy
- Poor radical prostatectomy candidates
- Outcome is stage dependent; lower-stage disease patients have better survival.
- Relapsed disease after prostatectomy
- Metastatic disease pain management

Conformal and Intensity-Modulated Radiation Therapy

- Conformal—Higher doses of radiation therapy are delivered more precisely to target area with less damage to normal surrounding structures and tissues.
- Intensity-modulated—Beam altered to deliver even more precise radiation to target tissue at a higher dose. Reduces rectal toxicity but may not reduce urinary tract toxicity.

External Beam Radiation Therapy Plus Hormonal Therapy[23, 24]

- Candidates include patients with higher-grade or higher-stage disease. Addition of hormonal therapy does improve control of local disease, freedom from distant metastases, and disease-free survival, all at 5 years.

Interstitial Brachytherapy[25–27]

Candidates include patients with
- T1 or T2 disease
- Older men with comorbidities
- Low Gleason score
- Low PSA
- May be combined with external beam radiation therapy

Systemic Radioisotopes[28]

- Candidates include patients with metastatic disease to the bone causing pain in multiple areas.
- May be used with external beam radiation therapy

Hormonal Therapy[29–30]

Candidates include patients
- Undergoing combined modality therapy with external beam radiation therapy
- With hormone-sensitive metastatic prostate cancer
- Monotherapy recommended as initial therapy.
- Retreatment with a second hormonal agent may be tried after the patient becomes refractory to the initial drug.

Bisphosphonates[31]

Candidates include patients
- On androgen suppressive therapy
- With metastatic hormone refractory prostate cancer

Chemotherapy[32–33]

- Candidates include patients with hormone-refractory metastatic prostate cancer and symptoms requiring palliation.
- Small survival advantage seen with docetaxel-based chemotherapy.

Clinical Trials

- A variety of trials are available for patients with all stages of prostate cancer.
- Refer to the National Cancer Institute's Physicians' Data Query service.

COMMON COMPLICATIONS OF TREATMENT

Surgical Complications Include[34]

- Urinary incontinence
- Urethral stricture
- Impotence
- Anesthesia and surgical complications
- Increased in patients older than 75
- Mortality rate—2% at 30 days
- Cardiovascular morbidity 8%

Radiation Complications Include

- Acute cystitis, proctitis, and enteritis
- Impotence
- Incontinence
- Frequent bowel movements
- Painful hemorrhoids
- Strictures

Hormonal Therapy Complications

Drug dependent but include
- Psychological effects
- Loss of libido
- Hot flashes
- Impotence
- Osteoporosis
- Gynecomastia and breast tenderness

- Tumor flare
- Diarrhea, nausea
- Liver toxicity
- Loss of muscle mass

Chemotherapy Complications

- Schedule, drug, and dose dependent
- Fatigue
- Anemia, leukopenia, and thrombocytopenia
- Nausea and vomiting
- Hair loss
- Phlebitis
- Thrombotic events, cardiovascular events
- Neutropenic fever

TREATMENT SELECTION FOR THE INDIVIDUAL PATIENT

- Each patient may have a number of treatment options available for his specific age, stage, expected survival, tumor factors, concurrent medical problems, patient preference, and acceptable side effect profile.
- Risks versus benefits of treatment must be determined for each patient.
- See **Table 6–1** for summary of treatment options.

TABLE 6–1 Summary of Treatment Options

Stage	TNM	WHO grade	Treatment Options for Each Stage
I	T1a N0 M0	1	1. Watchful waiting 2. Definitive treatment
II	T1 a N0 M0 T1 b N0 M0 T1 c N0 M0 T2 N0 M0	2, 3 Any Any Any	1. Radical prostatectomy 2. External beam radiation therapy 3. Interstitial brachytherapy 4. Watchful waiting 5. Cryosurgery
III	T3 N0 M0 T3 NX M0	Any	1. External beam radiation + hormonal therapy 2. External beam radiation therapy 3. Hormonal therapy 4. Radical prostatectomy (rarely) 5. Watchful waiting
IV	T4 N0 M0 Any T N1 M0 Any T any N M1	Any	1. Hormonal therapy 2. External beam radiation therapy (M0 only) 3. Palliative radiation therapy 4. Systemic radioisotopes for bone pain 5. Watchful waiting 6. Chemotherapy for hormone-refractory disease 7. Second-line hormonal therapy

WHO, World Health Organization.
Source: Adapted from Tester W, Mizrachi A, Brouch MD. Treatment decision making. In: Held-Warmkessel, J., ed. *Contemporary Issues in Prostate Cancer: A Nursing Perspective* (2nd ed). Sudbury, MA: Jones and Bartlett, 2006, 126–150.

PSYCHOSOCIAL ISSUES[35-45]

- Profound impact on individual, spouse, and family
- Wide range of reactions may occur.
- Psychological distress may impair decision making.
- Spiritual distress may also be a concern.
- Many patients are older but have concerns and problems that are different from younger men with prostate cancer that may include
  - Loss of income, limited resources
  - Loss of role identity
  - Loss of spouse/family
  - Loss of physiologic function
  - Loss of psychological function
- Other medical problems/comorbidities
- Reduced social support
- Impact on body image—masculinity, physical self, identity
- Impact of treatment-related complications—incontinence, impotence, bowel problems
- Self-imposed social isolation is related to complications.
- Constitutional symptoms contribute to reduced quality of life.
- Impact of drug-related side effects—loss of libido, feminization
- Impact on family/spouse—Different methods of coping between family members may compound stress. Spouses of prostate cancer patients are significantly affected by the patients' diagnosis. Patients may have different goals from therapy than their spouses. Patients are more likely to sacrifice some quantity of life for quality of life.
- Impact of sexual dysfunction

NURSING ISSUES AND CONCERNS[46-56]

- Assessment of patient knowledge base and providing patient education regarding understanding of physician-provided information, clarification of misconceptions, provision of accurate information, and answering questions
- Providing written information to enhance learning process
- Allowing patient and spouse to verbalize concerns about cancer diagnosis, treatment options available and their impact on quality of life, complications, and their management
- Functioning as a patient advocate
- Completing a psychosocial assessment, assess coping styles, identifying areas of need and concern, making appropriate referrals to social worker and support groups
- Promoting communication of patient questions and concerns to physician, spouse, and family
- Therapeutic listening
- Using of American Cancer Society and National Cancer Institute patient information
- Educating the patient/spouse about treatment-related complications, incidence, potential benefit, self-care of incontinence, and management of other complications
- Addressing sexual concerns with education and appropriate referrals for counseling
- Providing information of reliable health-related Web sites

- Providing symptom management information and patient education on self-care of treatment-related side effects.

References

1. Corral DA, Bahnson RR. Survival of men with clinically localized prostate cancer detected in the eighth decade of life. *J Urol.* 1994;152:1326–1329.
2. Zincke H, Bergstralh EJ, Blute ML, et al. Radical prostatectomy for clinically localized prostate cancer: long-term results of 1,143 patients from a single institution. *J Clin Oncol.* 1994;12:2254–2263.
3. Satariano WA, Ragland KE, Van Den Eeden SK. Cause of death in men diagnosed with prostate carcinoma. *Cancer.* 1998;83:1180–1188.
4. Helgesen F, Holmberg L, Johansson JE, et al. Trends in prostate cancer survival in Sweden, 1960 through 1988: evidence of increasing diagnosis of nonlethal tumors. *J Natl Cancer Instit.* 1996;88:1216–1221.
5. Vijayakumar S, Vaida F, Weichselbaum R, Hellman S. Race and the Will Rogers phenomenon in prostate cancer. *Cancer J Sci Am.* 1998;4:27–34.
6. Amling CL, Blute ML, Lerner S, et al. Influence of prostate-specific antigen testing on the spectrum of patients with prostate cancer undergoing radical prostatectomy at a large referral practice. *Mayo Clin Proc.* 1998;73:401–406.
7. Schuessler WW, Pharand D, Vancaillie TG. Laparoscopic standard pelvic node dissection for carcinoma of the prostate: is it accurate? *J Urol.* 1993;150:898–901.
8. Stone NN, Stock RG, Unger P. Indications for seminal vesicle biopsy and laparoscopic pelvic lymph node dissection in men with localized carcinoma of the prostate. *J Urol.* 1995;154:1392–1396.
9. Oesterling JE, Brendler CB, Epstein JI, et al. Correlation of clinical stage, serum prostatic acid phosphatase and preoperative Gleason grade with final pathological stage in 275 patients with clinically localized adenocarcinoma of the prostate. *J Urol.* 1987;138:92–98.
10. Albertsen PC, Fryback DG, Storer BE, et al. Long-term survival among men with conservatively treated localized prostate cancer. *JAMA.* 1995;274:626–631.
11. Bianco FJ, Wood DP, Cher ML. Ten-year survival after radical prostatectomy: specimen Gleason score is the predictor in organ-confined prostate cancer. *Clin Prostate Cancer.* 2003;1:242–247.
12. Lieber MM. Pathological stage C (pT3) prostate cancer treated by radical prostatectomy: clinical implications of DNA ploidy analysis. *Semin Urol.* 1990;8:219–224.
13. Rogers CG, Khan MA, Craig Miller M, et al. Natural history of disease progression in patients who fail to achieve an undetectable prostate-specific antigen level after undergoing radical prostatectomy. *Cancer.* 2004;101:2549–2556.
14. American Society for Therapeutic Radiology and Oncology Consensus Panel. Consensus statement: guidelines for PSA following radiation therapy. *Int J Radiat Oncol Biol Phys.* 1997;37:1035–1041.
15. Chodak GW, Thisted RA, Gerber GS, et al. Results of conservative management of clinically localized prostate cancer. *N Engl J Med.* 1994;330:242–248.
16. Johansson JE, Holmberg L, Johansson S, et al. Fifteen-year survival in prostate cancer: a prospective, population-based study in Sweden. *JAMA.* 1997;277:467–471.
17. Trabulsi EJ, Guillonneau B. Laparoscopic radical prostatectomy. *J Urol.* 2005;173:1072–1079.
18. Perez CA, Michalski JM, Baglan K, et al. Radiation therapy for increasing prostate-specific antigen levels after radical prostatectomy. *Clin Prostate Cancer.* 2003;1:235–241.

19. Duncan W, Warde P, Catton CN, et al. Carcinoma of the prostate: results of radical radiotherapy (1970–1985). *Int J Radiat Oncol Biol Phys.* 1993;26:203–210.
20. Hanks GE. Conformal radiotherapy for prostate cancer. *Ann Med.* 2000;32:57–63.
21. Jani AB, Roeske JC, Rash C. Intensity-modulated radiation therapy for prostate cancer. *Clin Prostate Cancer.* 2003;2:98–105.
22. Zelefsky MJ, Fuks Z, Hunt M, et al. High-dose radiation delivered by intensity modulated conformal radiotherapy improves the outcome of localized prostate cancer. *J Urol.* 2001;166:876–881.
23. Pilepich MV, Caplan R, Byhardt RW, et al. Phase III trial of androgen suppression using goserelin in unfavorable-prognosis carcinoma of the prostate treated with definitive radiotherapy. *J Clin Oncol.* 1997;15:1013–1021.
24. Bolla M, Gonzalez D, Warde P, et al. Improved survival in patients with locally advanced prostate cancer treated with radiotherapy and goserelin. *N Engl J Med.* 1997;337:295–300.
25. Ragde H, Blasko JC, Grimm PD, et al. Interstitial iodine-125 radiation without adjuvant therapy in the treatment of clinically localized prostate carcinoma. *Cancer.* 1997;80:442–453.
26. Sharkey J, Chovnick SD, Behar RJ, et al. Out-patient ultrasound-guided palladium 103 brachytherapy for localized adenocarcinoma of the prostate: a preliminary report of 434 patients. *Urology.* 1998;51:796–803.
27. Critz FA, Levinson AK, Williams WH, et al. Simultaneous radiotherapy for prostate cancer: I–125 prostate implant followed by external beam radiotherapy. *Cancer J Sci Am.* 1998;4:359–363.
28. Porter AT, McEwan AJ, Powe JE, et al. Results of a randomized phase-III trial to evaluate the efficacy of strontium-89 adjuvant to local field external beam irradiation in the management of endocrine-resistant metastatic prostate cancer. *Int J Radiat Oncol Biol Phys.* 1993;25:805–813.
29. Loblow DA, Mendelson DS, Talcott JA, et al. American Society of Clinical Oncology recommendations for the initial hormonal management of androgen-sensitive, metastatic, recurrent, or progressive prostate cancer. *J Clin Oncol.* 2004;22: 2927–2941.
30. Small EJ, Vogelzang NJ. Second-line hormonal therapy for advanced prostate cancer: a shifting paradigm. *J Clin Oncol.* 1997;15:382–388.
31. Smith MR, McGovern FJ, Zietman AL, et al. Pamidronate to prevent bone loss during androgen-deprivation therapy for prostate cancer. *N Engl J Med.* 2001;345: 948–955.
32. Tannock IF, de Wit R, Berry WR, et al. Docetaxel plus prednisone or mitoxantrone plus prednisone for advanced prostate cancer. *N Engl J Med.* 2004;351:1502–1512.
33. Petrylak DP, Tangen C, Hussain M, et al. Docetaxel and estramustine compared with mitoxantrone and prednisone for advanced refractory prostate cancer *N Engl J Med.* 2004;351:1513–1520.
34. Lu-Yao GL, McLerran D, Wasson J, et al. An assessment of radical prostatectomy: time trends, geographic variation, and outcomes. *JAMA.* 1993;269:2633–2636.
35. Davison BJ, Degner LF. Empowerment of men newly diagnosed with prostate cancer. *Cancer Nurs.* 1997;20:187–196.
36. McCray ND. Psychosocial and quality-of-life issues. In: Otto SE, ed. *Oncology Nursing.* 2nd ed. St. Louis, Mo: CV Mosby; 1997:817–834.
37. Engelking C. Comfort issues in geriatric oncology. *Semin Oncol Nurs.* 1988;4: 198–207.

38. O'Connor L, Blesch KS. Life cycle issues affecting cancer rehabilitation. *Semin Oncol Nurs.* 1992;8:174–185.
39. Barsevick AM, Much J, Sweeney C. Psychosocial responses to cancer. In: Groenwald MH, Frogge M, Goodman M, Yarbro CH, eds. *Cancer Nursing: Principles and Practice.* 4th ed. Sudbury, Mass: Jones and Bartlett; 1997:1393–1410.
40. Shell JA, Smith CK. Sexuality and the older person with cancer. *Oncol Nurs Forum.* 1994;21:553–558.
41. Burt K. The effects of cancer on body image and sexuality. *Nurs Times.* 1995;91:36–37.
42. Ofman U. Preservation of function in genitourinary cancers: psychosexual and psychosocial issues. *Cancer Invest.* 1995;13:125–131.
43. Northouse LL, Peters-Golden H. Cancer and the family: strategies to assist spouses. *Semin Oncol Nurs.* 1993;9:74–82.
44. Ofman U. Psychosocial and sexual implications of genitourinary cancers. *Semin Oncol Nurs.* 1993;9:286–292.
45. Lewis FM. Psychosocial transitions and the family's work in adjusting to cancer. *Semin Oncol Nurs.* 1993;9:127–129.
46. O'Rourke ME, Germino BB. Prostate cancer treatment decisions: a focus group exploration. *Oncol Nurs Forum.* 1998;25:97–104.
47. Davison BJ, Degner LF, Morgan TR. Information and decision-making preferences of men with prostate cancer. *Oncol Nurs Forum.* 1995;22:1401–1408.
48. Anderson B. Sexual functioning morbidity among cancer survivors. *Cancer.* 1985;55:1835–1842.
49. Fisher SG. The psychosexual effects of cancer and cancer treatment. *Oncol Nurs Forum.* 1983;10:63–67.
50. Peters-Golden H. Breast cancer: varied perceptions of social support in the illness experience. *Soc Sci Med.* 1982;16:463–491.
51. Singer PA, Tasch ES, Stocking C, et al. Sex or survival: trade-offs between quality and quantity of life. *J Clin Oncol.* 1991;9:328–334.
52. Volk RJ, Cantor SB, Cass AR, et al. Preferences of husbands and wives for outcomes of prostate cancer screening and treatment. *J Gen Intern Med.* 2004;19:339–348.
53. Mellon S, Northouse LL. Family survivorship and quality of life following a cancer diagnosis. *Research in Nursing Health.* 2001;24:446–459.
54. Calabrese D. Prostate cancer in older men. *Urol Nurs.* 2004;24:258–264,268–269.
55. Manyak M, Calabrese DA. Improving men's health: innovations in the treatment of prostate cancer. Medscape Web site. Available at: http://www.medscape.com/viewprogram/2440_index. Accessed November 30, 2004.
56. Meade-D'Alisera P, Saad F, Weingard KK. The management of complications related to prostate cancer and evolving role for nurses. Medscape Web site. Available at http://www.medscape.com/viewprogram/2133_index. Accessed November 30, 2004.

Chapter 7

Expectant Management: The Art and Science of Watchful Waiting

INTRODUCTION[1-3]
- Expectant management = watchful waiting = surveillance therapy = observation
- Therapy is the management of prostate cancer by initial assessment and workup with treatment administered if the cancer progresses to produce symptoms that bother the patient.
- Time to disease progression varies among different patients, but average is as long as 10 years
- Routine monitoring by digital rectal examination (DRE) and measurement of serum prostate-specific antigen (PSA) levels is performed.

RATIONALE FOR EXPECTANT MANAGEMENT[3-11]
- Incidence of prostate cancer is significantly higher than the death rate from the disease.
- Death rate is greater for dying with a prostate cancer diagnosis than from the prostate cancer as the cause of death.
- Lifetime risk of prostate cancer diagnosis is 10%.
- Lifetime risk of prostate cancer as a cause of death is 3%.
- Slow rate of tumor growth
- Approach may not be appropriate for African-American men with their higher incidence rate, more aggressive disease, and poorer survival rates.
- Tumors detected by PSA screening may be clinically insignificant and may not produce future morbidity for the patient.
- Treatment may detract from quality of life by producing distressing side effects, such as incontinence and impotence.
- Treatment may not result in more than a small gain (0.4–3 years) in life span.
- Watchful waiting has been used in Europe for over 30 years.
- Several published articles report similar survival at 10 and 15 years for men using this method. Many of the reports, however, are retrospective.
- No prospective randomized clinical trials demonstrating treatment is superior. Results of the Prostate Intervention Versus Observation Trial (PIVOT) and those being done in Europe will answer many questions and concerns about watchful waiting.
- Overall survival of patients on watchful waiting is 34–72% at 10 years.

RATIONALE AGAINST EXPECTANT MANAGEMENT [11, 13-17]
- Treatment with radical prostatectomy or radiation may cure the patient.
- Untreated prostate cancer may produce symptoms similar to treatment.
- Treatment may reduce psychological stress.
- Treatment may lower the risk of metastases and need for future treatment.
- May take 10–15 years to see impact of treatment versus watchful waiting.

- Patients may develop metastases after 10 years.
- May not be appropriate therapy for younger men with small tumors.
- Prostate cancer is a major health problem; second leading cause of cancer-related death.
- Cost, in terms of patient quality of life (QOL) is high when disease progresses.

THERAPEUTIC GOAL OF EXPECTANT MANAGEMENT [18-20]

- Avoid treatment-related complications in early stage cancer.
- Promote QOL.
- Avoid detracting from patient survival.
- No research exists to support these goals.
- May detract from QOL because of emotional issues around watchful waiting that require more research
- Minimal nursing literature on quality of life in patients using watchful waiting
- Patients may have worse general health.
- Patients may have more emotional issues with watchful waiting, such as anxiety.

PATIENT ELIGIBILITY CRITERIA [21-23]

- Patient life expectancy is $\leq$ 10 years due to age or comorbidities.
- Asymptomatic patients with advanced incurable disease
- Favorable pathology—Gleason score $<$ 7, low PSA density (0.10–0.15), less than three core biopsy specimens with cancer present or $<$ 50% cancer in each core biopsy specimen
- PSA $<$ 10 ng/mL
- Negative DRE
- Patient preference/spouse preference
- Ability to tolerate uncertainty
- NCCN guidelines[23] suggest that asymptomatic patients with these criteria may be watchful waiting candidates.
- Gleason score $\leq$ 7 and life expectancy $\leq$ 5 years
- Patients with T1–T2 disease, Gleason score 2–6, PSA $\leq$10, and life expectancy $\leq$ 10 years

PATIENT AND PARTNER VIEWS OF THE EXPECTANT
MANAGEMENT OPTION[24-31]

- May be perceived negatively by Americans.
- Survival difficult to predict.
- Patients tend to expect to live longer than is realistic.
- Little research on patient/spouse/partner views on watchful waiting; more research is needed.
- May be perceived as no intervention
- Active treatment may prevent recurrence and metastases.
- Active treatment viewed more favorably by patient's spouse or partner as method of improving patient's survival despite patient's concern about complications.
- Patients and spouses may feel that they have already waited enough already and do not want to wait anymore for definitive treatment.
- Patients may delay treatment hoping for better treatment than that currently available.

- Family experience with cancer and cancer therapy
- Social and cultural influences including the patient's perceptions of the physician and information-gathering processes
- Role models and public figures may influence patient's perceptions.

PROTOCOL FOR EXPECTANT MANAGEMENT [23, 32]

NCCN Guidelines [23]

- For patients with expected survival < 10 years, clinical exam every 6–12 months with PSA and DRE. In 1-year postdiagnosis, repeat prostate biopsy.
- For patients with expected survival > 10 years, clinical exam every 6 months with PSA and DRE. In 1-year postdiagnosis, repeat prostate biopsy.
- For patients with progressive disease, treatment may be appropriate.

Option One

For men with < 10- to 15-year expected lifespan with normal age-specific PSA
- Assessments would include DRE and PSA every 3 months for 1 year and then every 6–12 months with PSA drawn prior to clinical exam.
- Abnormal DRE or increase in PSA—restaging diagnostic studies including bone scan and transrectal ultrasonography (TRUS)-guided biopsies
- Treatment can be considered in presence of disease progression.

Option Two

PSA, DRE, and TRUS every 4–6 months
- Research is needed in this area to reduce the uncertainty involved in the use of watchful waiting, to fully describe the appropriate methodology of watchful waiting, and to develop research-based watchful waiting medical care and practice.

Monitoring PSA Velocity

A velocity of 2.0 ng/mL/year is an independent predictor of death from prostate cancer.[32]
- Patients likely to need treatment[33]—age < 65, initial PSA value > 10 ng/mL, clinical stage > T1

WHEN SHOULD TREATMENT BE PURSUED? [1, 23]

- Development of troublesome symptoms—consider hormonal therapy
- Surgery or radiation therapy for patients eligible for these modalities
- For patients not eligible for surgery or radiation therapy, hormonal therapy may be an option.
- PSA elevations
- Increased size of tumor
- Increased Gleason score on biopsy

NURSING MANAGEMENT OF PATIENTS CHOOSING THE EXPECTANT MANAGEMENT OPTION

Education of patient and partner about need to maintain schedule of appointments for PSA, DRE, and physical examination
- Have PSA drawn at the same laboratory prior to office visit so results are available for discussion with physician.
- Symptoms to report

Assessment of QOL parameters
Determination of symptom impact on QOL

PSYCHOEDUCATIONAL INTERVENTIONS TO MINIMIZE UNCERTAINTY[26, 34-38]

- Assist patient to deal with uncertainty with education and support.
- The problem of uncertainty of outcome when using watchful waiting as treatment option
- Uncertainty may result in other psychosocial problems such as depression and emotional distress.
- Monitor patient for difficulty with adjusting to watchful waiting
- Research needed in methods of assisting patients and spouses to deal with the uncertainty and to reduce the perceived negativity of watchful waiting/expectant management
- Psychosocial interventions may be useful, such as reframing, social comparison, ignoring the cancer, patient's focusing on the positive aspects of his situation in comparison with others
- Some patients may use CAM therapies.
- Use of spiritual support and support groups may be helpful.
- Awareness of cultural and ethnic concerns and differences
- Awareness of nonsynchronous adaptation by patient and spouse to watchful waiting
- Address patient and spouse individual concerns, answering questions, providing accurate information, encouraging verbalization, and providing education in the management of uncertainty.
- Understand that there may be regional, cultural, and physician differences in the use of watchful waiting.
- Internet sties may contain inaccurate information.
- Each reevaluation period may precipitate anxiety and uncertainty.

References

1. Adolfsson J. Deferred treatment for clinically localized prostate cancer. *Eur J Surg Oncol.* 1995;21:333–340.
2. Madsen PO, Graversen P, Gasser TC, et al. Treatment of localized prostate cancer. Radical prostatectomy versus placebo: a 15-year follow-up. *Scand J Urol Nephrol Suppl.* 1988;100:95–100.
3. Palmer JS, Chodak G. Defining the role of surveillance in the management of localized prostate cancer. *Urol Clin North Am.* 1996;23:551–556.
4. Steinberg GD, Bales GT, Bredler CB. An analysis of watchful waiting for clinically localized prostate cancer. *J Urol.* 1998;159:1431–1436.
5. Landis SH, Murray T, Bolden S, et al. Cancer statistics, 1999. *CA Cancer J Clin.* 1999;49:8–31.
6. Wilt TJ. Prostate cancer screening: practice what the evidence preaches. *Am J Med.* 1998;104:602–604.
7. Collins MM, Ransohoff DF, Barry MJ. Early detection of prostate cancer. Serendipity strikes again. *JAMA.* 1997;278:1516–1519.
8. American College of Physicians. Clinical Guideline: Part III. Screening for prostate cancer. *Ann Intern Med.* 1997;126:480–484.
9. Johansson JE, Holmberg L, Johansson S, et al. Fifteen-year survival in prostate cancer: results and identification of high-risk patient population. *JAMA.* 1997;277: 467–471.

10. Adolfsson J, Carstensen J, Lowhagen T. Deferred treatment in clinically localised prostate carcinoma. *Br J Urol.* 1992;69:183–187.
11. Aus G, Hugosson J, Norlen L. Long-term survival and mortality in prostate cancer treated with noncurative intent. *J Urol.* 1995;154:460–465.
12. Goodman CM, Busttil A, Chisholm GD. Age, size, and grade of tumor predict prognosis in incidentally diagnosed carcinoma of the prostate. *Br J Urol.* 1988;62: 576–580.
13. Small EJ. Prostate cancer. *Curr Opin Oncol.* 1997;9:277–286.
14. Brausi M, Palladin PD, Latini A. "Watchful waiting" for clinically localized prostate cancer: Long-term results [abstract]. *Eur Oncol.* 1996;30(suppl 2):225.
15. McLaren DB, McKenzie M, Duncan G, Pickles T. Watchful waiting or watchful progression? Prostate-specific antigen doubling times and clinical behavior in patients with early untreated prostate carcinoma. *Cancer.* 1998;82:342–348.
16. Holmberg L, Bill-Axelson K, Helgesen F, et al. A randomized trial comparing radical prostatectomy with watchful waiting in early prostate cancer. *N Engl J Med.* 2002;347:781–796.
17. Hugosson J, Aus G, Norlen L. Surveillance is not a viable and appropriate treatment option in the management of localized prostate cancer. *Urol Clin North Am.* 1996;23:557–573.
18. Litwin MS, Hays RD, Fink A, et al. Quality of life and treatment outcomes in men treated for localized prostate cancer. *JAMA.* 1995;273:129–135.
19. Galbraith ME, Ramirez JM, Pedro LW. Quality of life, health outcomes, and identity for patients with prostate cancer in five different treatment groups. *Oncol Nurs Forum.* 2001;28:55–60.
20. Wallace M. Uncertainty and quality of life of older men who undergo watchful waiting for prostate cancer. *Oncol Nurs Forum.* 2003;30:303–309.
21. Nam R, Klotz IH, Jewett MAS, et al. Prostate-specific antigen velocity as a measure of the natural history of prostate cancer: identification of a rapid riser subset. *Br J Urol.* 1998;81:100–104.
22. Walsh PC, Brooks, JD. The Swedish cancer paradox. *JAMA.* 1997;277:497–498.
23. Scherr D, Swindle PW, Scardino PT. National Comprehensive Cancer Network guidelines for the management of prostate cancer. *Urology.* 2003;61(suppl 1):14–21.
24. O'Rourke ME, Germino BB. Prostate cancer treatment selection: a focus group exploration. *Oncol Nurs Forum.* 1998;25:97–103.
25. Mazur DJ, Merz JF. How older patients' treatment preferences are influenced by disclosures about therapeutic uncertainty: surgery versus expectant management for localized prostate cancer. *J Am Geriatr Soc.* 1996;44:934–937.
26. O'Rourke ME. Prostate cancer treatment selection: the family decision process [dissertation]. University of North Carolina, Chapel Hill; 1997.
27. O'Rourke ME, Germino BB. Spousal caregiving across the prostate cancer trajectory. *Quality Life: Nurs Challenge.* 1998;6:66–72.
28. Volk RJ, Cantor SB, Spann SJ, et al. Preferences of husbands and wives for prostate cancer screening. *Arch Fam Med.* 1997;6:72–76.
29. Weeks JC, Cook EF, O'Day SJ, et al. Relationship between cancer patients' predictions of prognosis and their treatment preferences. *JAMA.* 1998;279:1709–1714.
30. Mazur DJ, Merz JF. Older patients' willingness to trade off urologic adverse outcomes for a better chance at five-year survival in the clinical setting of prostate cancer. *J Am Geriatr Soc.* 1995;43:979–984.

31. Nattinger AB, Hoffman RG, Howell-Pelz A, Goodwin JS. Effect of Nancy Reagan's mastectomy on choice of surgery for breast cancer by US women. *JAMA*. 1998;279:762–766.
32. D'Amci AV, Chen MH, Roehl KA, et al. Preoperative PSA velocity and the risk of death from prostate cancer after radical prostatectomy. *N Engl J Med*. 2004;351:125–135.
33. Wu H, Moul JW, Wu HY, et al. Watchful waiting and factors predictive of secondary treatment of localized prostate cancer. *J Urol*. 2004;171:1111–1116.
34. Mishel MH, Germino BB, Belyea M, et al. Predictors of emotional distress in African-American men with prostate cancer and African-American women with breast cancer. The experience of uncertainty in older Caucasian and African-American cancer patients. Symposium presented at the 11th annual conference of the Southern Nursing Research Society. Norfolk, Va, 1997.
35. Germino BB, Michel MH, Ware A, et al. Uncertainty in prostate cancer: ethnic and family patterns. *Cancer Pract*. 1998;6:107–113.
36. Bailey DE, Mishel MH. Uncertainty management strategies for men electing watchful waiting as a treatment option for prostate cancer [abstract 156]. *Oncol Nurs Forum*. 1997;24:326.
37. Hedestig O, Sandman PO, Widmark A. Living with untreated localized prostate cancer: a qualitative analysis of patient narratives. *Cancer Nurs*. 2003;26:55–60.
38. Taylor SE, Bunk BP, Collins RL, Reed GM. Social comparison and affiliation under threat. In: Montada L, Fillip SH, Lerner MJ, eds. *Life Crises and Experiences of Loss in Adulthood*. Hillsdale, N.J.: Erlbaum; 1992:213–227.

Chapter 8
Surgery

INTRODUCTION

Uses for Surgical Interventions

- Diagnosis (biopsy)
- Staging
- Cure
- Symptom reduction and palliation
- See **Table 8–1** for standard of care for patients undergoing surgery for the treatment of prostate cancer.[1–3]

TRANSURETHRAL RESECTION OF THE PROSTATE (TURP)

Purpose of Surgical Procedure

- Used to relieve symptoms of bladder outlet obstruction (BOO) caused by the enlarging prostate tumor compressing the prostatic urethra or from tumor interfering with the normal function of the urinary sphincter.

BOO Symptoms [4–5]

- Urgency
- Frequency
- Nocturia
- Retention
- Dysuria
- Overflow incontinence
- Lower abdominal pain

Candidates [6]

- Patients > 70
- Life expectancy < 10 years

TURP is also used to treat benign prostatic hyperplasia (BPH). If an unsuspected cancer is found on tissue pathology, the stage is either T1, T1a, or T1b.[7] These patients may be eligible for additional surgical resection.

Procedure[1, 7, 8]

- Anesthesia used—general or spinal
- Position—lithotomy
- Uses electrocautery via transurethral resectoscope to remove chips of anterior, posterior, and lateral areas of prostate
- Continuous bladder irrigation (CBI) runs during the procedure to remove chips of tissue and blood
- Resected chips are sent to pathology for analysis.
- A three-way indwelling urinary drainage catheter with a 30 mL balloon is placed and taped to the patient's thigh with tension to help control bleeding in the resected prostatic fossa.

TABLE 8-1 Standard of Care for Patient's Undergoing Surgery for Treatment of Prostate Cancer

NURSING DIAGNOSIS: Knowledge deficit regarding surgery

EXPECTED OUTCOME: Patient will verbalize understanding of perioperative course.

NURSING INTERVENTIONS:

1. Assess patient's readiness to learn, learning preferences, barriers to teaching, and who to include in teaching.
2. Assess patient's knowledge of prostate cancer and planned procedure.
3. Educate on the following: • Need for bowel preparation • NPO after midnight except clear liquids up to 6 hours prior to surgery • Coughing and deep breathing • Incentive spirometry • Antiembolism or compression stocking • Early ambulation • Care of catheters and drains • Bladder spasms • Pain management • Incision • Increased fluid intake after TURP • No straining with bowel movement • Signs and symptoms of infection
4. Include family in teaching and obtain feedback.

NURSING DIAGNOSIS: Altered urinary elimination

EXPECTED OUTCOME: Catheter will remain patent, and patient will maintain urinary output of at least 30 cc/hour.

NURSING INTERVENTIONS:

1. Assess bladder for distention by palpating bladder above pubic symphysis.
2. Assess patency of catheter.
3. Keep catheter taped securely at all times.
4. Maintain accurate intake and output every shift.
5. Empty urinary drainage bag when two thirds full to keep bladder from becoming distended.
6. Adjust rate of continuous bladder irrigation (CBI) as needed to keep urine clear.
7. Do not allow CBI bags to become empty.
8. Manually irrigate catheter with normal saline as needed to remove clots, but do not forcefully irrigate.
9. Encourage fluid intake to 2–3 L/day.
10. Maintain IV therapy at prescribed rate.
11. Educate on the following: • Care for catheter. • Manage leg and night drainage bags. • Secure catheter at all times. • Keep drainage bag below level of bladder. • Monitor for signs and symptoms of obstruction and urinary tract infections and notify physician if they occur.
12. Discontinue catheter as ordered. Notify physician if patient does not void within 8 hours.

NURSING DIAGNOSIS: Risk for fluid and electrolyte imbalance

EXPECTED OUTCOME: Patient will maintain a urinary output of at least 30 cc/hour. Electrolytes will be within normal parameters.

NURSING INTERVENTIONS:

1. Monitor electrolytes, BUN, and creatinine. Report abnormal values to physician.
2. Monitor for changes in renal and cardiac function.
3. Monitor intake and output, including hydration status (i.e., edema). Report imbalances to physician.

NPO, nothing by mouth; TURP, transurethral resection of the prostate.

continues

TABLE 8–1 Standard of Care for Patient's Undergoing Surgery for Treatment of Prostate Cancer,[1-3] continued

4. Maintain IV therapy as prescribed.

5. Report any changes in mental status or vital signs to physician. Assess for nausea, vomiting, malaise, decreased level of consciousness, and presence of tremors, visual disturbances, or headaches.

6. Place patient on fall/injury precautions.

NURSING DIAGNOSIS: Bleeding related to surgery

EXPECTED OUTCOME: Patient will remain hemodynamically stable, as evidenced by no overt signs of bleeding and stable vital signs.

NURSING INTERVENTIONS:

1. Monitor hemoglobin and hematocrit. Notify physician of decrease in hemoglobin of 1 g or greater.

2. Assess dressing for signs of bleeding.

3. Monitor vital signs for tachycardia and hypotension.

4. Assess catheter, drains, and nasogastric tube for signs of bleeding.

5. Assess for signs of hypoxia: • Pulse oximetry • Lethargy • Anxiety • Restlessness • Change in mental status

6. If in use, maintain traction on catheter to control venous bleeding.

7. Monitor for bladder distention.

8. Discontinue catheter with physician order only.

NURSING DIAGNOSIS: Risk for thrombophlebitis and pulmonary embolism

EXPECTED OUTCOME: Patient will not experience thrombophlebitis or pulmonary embolism.

NURSING INTERVENTIONS:

1. Assess patient for shortness of breath.

2. Assess patient's calf and arm for: • Pain • Redness • Edema • Warmth

3. Patient wears antiembolism stockings and compression devices when in bed.

4. Reinforce leg exercises as instructed preoperatively.

5. Ambulate patient on postoperative day 1.

6. Administer anticoagulants as prescribed.

NURSING DIAGNOSIS: Altered comfort related to pain and bladder spasm

EXPECTED OUTCOME: Patient will verbalize acceptable level of comfort.

NURSING INTERVENTIONS:

1. Assess quantity, quality, and duration of pain.

2. Assess for bladder distention, kinked tubing, and free flow of urine.

3. Assess security of catheter and retape as needed.

4. Administer narcotics for pain as prescribed.

5. Administer antispasmodics as prescribed.

6. Educate on the following: • Splint incision when getting in and out of bed and coughing and deep breathing. • Wear scrotal supporters if indicated. • Take sitz bath if indicated. • Nonpharmacologic methods for pain management (e.g., distraction, guided imagery).

NPO, nothing by mouth; TURP, transurethral resection of the prostate.

continues

TABLE 8-1 Standard of Care for Patient's Undergoing Surgery for Treatment of Prostate Cancer,[1-3] continued

NURSING DIAGNOSIS: Risk of infection related to surgery and indwelling catheter

EXPECTED OUTCOME: Patient will not experience a fever or other signs of infection.

NURSING INTERVENTIONS:

1. Assess for signs of infection and notify physician if present: • Fever $\geq$ 38.5°C • Redness, pain, swelling, and drainage from incision and drain sites • Cloudy or foul-smelling urine • Increase in white blood cell count • Tachycardia • Diaphoresis • Mental status changes • Change in breath sounds

2. Encourage coughing, deep breathing, and incentive spirometry every hour.

3. Perform catheter care twice a day with soap and water.

4. Use aseptic technique when emptying or changing drainage bag.

5. Obtain urine, blood, or other cultures as prescribed.

NURSING DIAGNOSIS: Risk of constipation as a result of narcotics and antispasmodics

EXPECTED OUTCOME: Patient will have easy bowel movement.

NURSING INTERVENTIONS:

1. Administer stool softeners and laxatives as prescribed.

2. Encourage patient to drink at least 2–3 L of fluid a day.

3. Educate patient not to strain when moving bowels.

4. Ambulate once on postoperative day 1 and then a least twice a day.

5. Increase fiber in diet.

NURSING DIAGNOSIS: Incontinence resulting from surgery

EXPECTED OUTCOME: Patient will be able to manage incontinence.

NURSING INTERVENTIONS:

1. After removal of indwelling catheter, educate on measures to assist in alleviating incontinence: • Modification in dietary habits and fluid intake • Timed voiding • Kegel exercises • Behavior modification • Incontinence devices • Possible surgical interventions and/or pharmacologic interventions

2. Educate on personal hygiene.

NURSING DIAGNOSIS: Body image disturbance related to cancer diagnosis and surgery

EXPECTED OUTCOME: Patient and family will adapt to altered body image.

NURSING INTERVENTIONS:

1. Assess ability to adjust to altered body image.

2. Provide opportunities for patient and family to discuss feelings of altered body image.

3. Emphasize that disease and surgery have no affect on patient's masculinity.

4. Reassure patient of ability to continue roles and relationships with family and friends.

5. If patient wishes, arrange for him to talk with someone who has had surgery for prostate cancer.

6. Refer patient and family to support or self-help group or psychosocial health care team members if appropriate.

NPO, nothing by mouth; TURP, transurethral resection of the prostate.

Source: Mason, TM. Surgery. In: Held-Warmkessel, J., ed. *Contemporary Issues in Prostate Cancer: A Nursing Perspective* (2nd ed). Jones and Bartlett Publishers, 2006, 166–182. Reprinted with permission by Jones and Bartlett Publishers.

- CBI continues to run for 24 hours to remove clots.
- May be done as an outpatient procedure, and the patient is discharged after voiding that is free of large clots or frank blood.

Preoperative Teaching Includes [9]

- Deep breathing, use of incentive spirometry (IS), early ambulation, indwelling urinary catheter until urine is clear, 2 L/day fluid intake, antispasmodics for bladder spasms, use of stool softeners to avoid straining on bowel movement, postoperative care, preoperative antibiotics
- Bladder spasms and urge to void may occur from the indwelling urinary catheter and its large balloon.[7-8]
- Stopping all medications with anticoagulant properties such as aspirin (10 days prior to surgery), warfarin (7 days prior to surgery) (a heparin drip is stopped 4 hours before surgery and restarted 30 minutes after surgery), herbs, vitamins, and nonsteroidal anti-inflammatory drugs 7–10 days before surgery

Monitor for Postoperative Complications

Respiratory compromise[9]
- Monitor patient for development of atelectasis, pneumonia, or pooled respiratory secretions.
- Monitor patient for cardiovascular complications, such as DVT or pulmonary embolus.
- Encourage deep breathing and use of IS.
- Coughing may cause bleeding.
- Early ambulation
- Q4H vital signs

Transurethral Resection (TUR) Syndrome
- Develops when large amounts of CBI is absorbed causing hypervolemia and hyponatremia; symptoms include changes in mental status and vision and cardiac and renal dysfunction.

Bleeding and Clot Retention[7]
- Monitor CBI, assess inflow and output every 30 minutes for retention.
- Keep tubing straight and unkinked to reduce risk of retention and bladder spasms.
- Keep catheter taped to thigh.
- Manually irrigate catheter to dislodge clots but never forcefully—call urologist
- Adjust flow rate of CBI to keep urine colorless to light pink.
- Monitor amount of bleeding; if heavy, call urologist.
- Bleeding may be venous (burgundy color) or arterial (bright red).
- Oral intake of 2 liters per day after IV fluids stopped

Urinary Tract Infection (UTI)
- Use strict aseptic technique; administer prescribed antibiotics.

Bladder Spasms
- Related to surgery, presence of catheter; administer antispasmodics and analgesics.
- Keep CBI running. Spasms may stop CBI flow.
- Monitor fluid balance.
- Measure intake and output (I&O).
- Administer intravenous fluids.
- Encourage oral fluids if patient is not nauseated or vomiting.

- Notify urologist if urine output < 30 mL/hour or if intake is greater than output, and assess for urinary retention.

Constipation and GI Side Effects

- Patients may develop constipation with straining, which increases the risk of bleeding and clot retention.
- Administer stool softeners.
- Educate patient to avoid constipation and straining and to use stool softeners for 6 weeks after surgery or longer.

Removal of Indwelling Urinary Catheter

- If urine is clear yellow to light pink, (urologist's discretion), remove only on order of urologist; monitor voiding after removal, as retention may occur from retained chips or clots or bladder atony.
- Catheter reinsertion may be necessary.

Discharge Planning

- Arrange home care if patient is discharged with a urinary catheter.

Discharge Teaching

- Educate the patient with urinary retention to call the urologist, as a catheter may need to be reinserted.
- Small clots and pieces of tissue may be present in the urine.
- Fluid intake of 2 liters/day unless contraindicated by medical comorbidity
- Care of catheter—see **Table 8–2**[10–11]

Long-Term TURP Complications[8, 12]

- Incontinence
- Impotence
- Urethral stricture
- Bladder neck contracture
- Retrograde ejaculation
- Repeat obstruction from enlarged prostate gland
- Educate patient as to signs and symptoms to report to urologist.

RADICAL PROSTATECTOMY[1, 13–17]

- Potentially curative surgical procedure
- Usage has increased with increased number of patients diagnosed with early disease due to PSA testing with an increase in 10-year biochemical disease-free survival.

Candidates—T1 or T2 Disease

- Good medical health status with no significant comorbidities
- Life expectancy > 10 years.
- PSA < 20 ng/mL
- Selected patients with T3 or N+ disease when treated with multimodality therapy.

Of patients undergoing radical retropubic prostatectomy (RRP), 20–60% have stage upgrades on pathology.

Procedure[1, 2, 14, 15, 18, 20, 21]

- Removal of entire prostate, prostatic capsule, seminal vesicles, part of bladder neck, reanastomosis of urethra, placement of indwelling urinary drainage catheter

TABLE 8–2 Guidelines for Urinary Catheter Care—Patient and Caregiver[10–11]

CLEANSING MEATUS AND CATHETER—at least twice a day and after bowel movement or per physician's order

1. Wash hands with soap and warm water at least 15 seconds.
2. Inspect meatus and surrounding tissue for inflammation, swelling, and drainage.
3. Using a clean washcloth, soap, and water, spread urethral meatus, cleanse around catheter in circular motion, then meatus and skin folds.
4. With another clean washcloth, soap, and water, clean 4 inches of length of catheter.
5. Reposition foreskin, if applicable.
6. Apply antibiotic ointment, if ordered, at meatus.
7. Dispose of cleaning supplies.
8. Wash hands.

CLEANSING DRAINAGE BAGS

1. After removal of leg bag or night drainage bag, fill with warm water and antibacterial soap. Shake gently and rinse.
2. A vinegar and water solution can also be used to help decrease odor: 1 cup vinegar to 2 quarts of water.
3. After cleansing, hang the bag from a shower curtain or rod to air dry.
4. Wash hands.

EMPTYING URINE (when two thirds full)

1. Wash hands with soap and water.
2. While not touching the drain port, turn the cap clockwise (or open clip) and drain into a collection container or directly into the toilet.
3. Turn cap counterclockwise to close (or close clip).
4. Wash hands.
5. If requested, record amount of urine drained in voiding diary.

CHANGING BAGS

1. Empty leg bag (as above).
2. Clamp catheter (can use a clothespin).
3. Wipe the connections between the catheter and leg bag with alcohol wipe.
4. Disconnect the leg bag from catheter, being careful not to pull on catheter.
5. Connect the night drainage bag to the catheter.
6. Unclamp the catheter.
7. Secure night drainage bag to thigh.
8. Clean leg bag (as above).
9. Wash hands.

When changing from night drainage bag to leg bag, empty the night drainage bag and follow the steps above.

Source: Mason, TM. Surgery. In: Held-Warmkessel, J., ed. *Contemporary Issues in Prostate Cancer: A Nursing Perspective* (2nd ed). Jones and Bartlett Publishers, 2006, 166–182. Reprinted with permission by Jones and Bartlett Publishers.

- Anesthesia—general or spinal
- Incision—retropubic (via a vertical abdominal incision with lymph node dissection) or perineal (via a perineal incision performed in lithotomy position, second incision needed to remove lymph nodes)
- Lymph node dissection is part of standard therapy.
- Lymph node dissection may not be done on some low risk for metastases patients, but then some patients with positive nodes will have disease left behind.

Nerve Sparing Procedure[21, 22]

- Nerves responsible for erectile function are left intact. One or both nerves may be left intact.
- This is not done if there is the risk of disease being left behind.
- Contraindications to nerve sparing procedure
  - T3c disease
  - Palpable apex of gland disease
  - Gleason score > 5
  - PSA > 20 ng/mL
  - Preexisting erectile dysfunction

Benefit of Retropubic Approach[13, 16, 21]

- Considered gold standard procedure
- Open lymph node dissection, nerve-sparing technique if patient is appropriate candidate
- Better hemostasis
- Better view of neurovascular bundles
- Wide excision can be done
- Only one excision needed to remove lymph nodes and prostate gland
- If lymph nodes contain metastatic disease, procedure is abandoned.

Benefit of Perineal Approach[13, 15, 16]

- Less blood loss, less pain, easier urethra reanastomosis
- Shorter length of stay
- Possibly fewer post-op complications

Disadvantages of Perineal Approach[13, 20, 23]

- Laparoscopic lymph node dissection or separate incision needed for lymph node dissection
- Higher risk of rectal injury and sexual dysfunction
- Patients with positive nodes on lymph node dissection can avoid additional surgical intervention.

Salvage Radical Prostatectomy[14, 24]

- May be an option for patients with local disease relapse after prior local therapy
- Risk of incontinence and erectile dysfunction high
- Risk of rectal damage
- Risk of need for cystectomy (rare)

Preoperative Teaching

- Bowel preparation, clear liquid diet, coughing and deep breathing, incentive spirometry, compression stockings, early ambulation, presence of urinary bladder catheter, nasogastric tube, surgical site drain(s), antibiotics, IV fluids, NPO status, postoperative course

Postoperative Management[1, 15, 25]

See **Table 8–1** and **Table 8–2**.
Indwelling urinary catheter care
- Keep taped securely in place at all times.
- Do not manipulate catheter.
- Keep tubing unkinked and straight.
- Assess patient for distention and retention.
- Wash urinary meatus twice daily with soap and water; teach patient how to perform self-care.
- Teach patient how to change from straight drainage to leg bag and to use straight drainage at night.
- Teach patient how to maintain cleanliness of bags and use of clean technique.
- Monitor fluid balance and I&O.
- Arrange home care for wound monitoring and continued education in self-care of urinary catheter.
- Do not remove catheter.

Monitor for postoperative complications such as
- Bleeding
- Thrombophlebitis
- Pulmonary embolus
- UTI and wound infection

Nursing Interventions

Immediate postoperative care
- Frequent vital signs, I&O, dressing monitoring
- Assess for internal bleeding: ↑ heart rate, ↓ blood pressure (BP).
- Assess for hypovolemia: ↓ BP, ↓ urine output (assess for retention).
- Assess for fluid overload and pulmonary embolus: ↑ respiratory rate.
- Assess for infection: ↑ temperature, drainage from wound.
- Assess for decreased urine output (< 30 mL/hour)—hourly I&O.
- Reinforce dressings, monitor wound.
- Empty drains; record volume.
- Apply antiembolism stockings, administer any prescribed anticoagulants.
- Administer IV fluids and prescribed antibiotics.
- Monitor for bladder spasms. Check for urinary retention and blocked catheter as causes.
- Pain management
- Encourage coughing, deep breathing, use of incentive spirometry, leg movements.
- Assess effect of analgesic regimen. Administer patient-controlled analgesia as prescribed. Encourage wound splinting prior to coughing, deep breathing, and movement.
- Administer antispasmodics.
- Assess bowel function; nasogastric tube to suction.
- Avoid anything per rectum; administer prescribed stool softeners, laxatives.

Postoperative day 1
- Nasogastric tube removed; clear liquid diet started
- Assess bowel sounds and patient's tolerance to diet.
- Promote ambulation.
- Continue coughing, deep breathing, incentive spirometry, antiembolism stockings, I&O, and volume of drainage.

- Monitor bowel function.
- See **Table 8-1** for standard of care.
- Arrange for home care services.
- Initiate patient education.

Care on post-op day #2 and beyond
- Advance diet as tolerated.
- Ambulation
- Ongoing care as above
- Drains removed 4–5 days post-op.

Post-op Patient Education[1, 15, 26]

- Notify urologist of signs and symptoms of infection, clot retention, bleeding, or leakage of urine.
- Care of indwelling urinary catheter
- Indwelling catheter left intact for 2–4 weeks
- Need to avoid constipation with stool softeners and laxatives
- No heavy moving or lifting, no strenuous activities for 4–6 weeks after surgery
- Care of drains if discharged with them left in place
  - Notify urologist if increased drainage or bleeding occur.
- Incontinence and dribbling after catheter removed should resolve in several months.
  - Use of incontinence devices
  - Skin care
  - Hygiene
  - Fluid monitoring and reducing evening intake
  - Frequent voiding
  - Kegel exercises may be started after catheter removed
- Sexuality issues
  - Retrograde ejaculation
  - Erectile dysfunction
- Pain management

Long-Term Complications

- Urinary incontinence
- Fecal incontinence
- Impotence
- Bladder neck contracture
- Urethral stricture
- Lymphedema
- Disease recurrence

CRYOABLATION OF THE PROSTATE

- Use of freezing temperatures to kill cancer cells[27]

Candidates[14, 16, 26–29]

- Patients with local or locally advanced disease
- Salvage therapy after local failure of prior therapy
- Older patients
- Patients with comorbidities
- May be used alone or with other local therapies and procedure can be repeated.
- Should be done as part of a clinical trial; procedure is investigational.

Procedure[8, 13, 18, 27, 28, 30]

- General anesthesia
- Lithotomy position
- Suprapubic catheter (SPC) placed and bladder filled with saline
- Urethral warming device placed
- Done with transrectal ultrasound guidance
- Probes inserted percutaneously via perineum into prostate
- Liquid nitrogen or other freezing gas runs into probes and freezes tissue. Necrosis occurs and necrotic tissue is removed by body via the urethra.

Preoperative Patient Education

- Bowel preparation, wound care, SPC care, and routine preoperative care (NPO, antiembolism stockings, antibiotics), stopping medications with anticoagulant properties, post-op course

Postoperative Care[1]

- Frequent vital signs, I&O, assess tube drainage, assess catheter tube patency, keep tubing straight, flush tube as needed to maintain patency, monitor color of urine, assess for infection, monitor wound for infection or bleeding, IV fluids, hygiene, pain management, soft diet, arrange for home care, ambulation

Discharge Patient Education[18, 31]

SPC care
- Clamping and unclamping SPC to perform postvoid residuals starts about 1 week after procedure.
- Washing around catheter with soap and water, apply dry sterile gauze, and attach leg bag during day and straight drainage bag at night.
- Notify urologist if unable to void after SPC removed.
- Home care for SPC removal after 7 days, depending on amount of postvoid residuals
- Catheter securement
- Skin care
- Catheter bag care
- Catheter irrigation

Perineal wound care
- Local care, sitz baths

Scrotal edema
- Ice and leg elevations

Other post-op care
- Pain management, bladder spasm management
- Fluid intake
- Avoiding constipation, no straining
- Patient education as to signs and symptoms of infection and other postprocedure complications

Complications[16, 23, 28–30]

- Urethral sloughing starts 4–6 weeks postprocedure and lasts about 8 weeks
- Urinary tract obstruction
- Fistulas
- Incontinence

- Impotence
- Bladder neck contractures
- Penile numbness
- Disease recurrence
- Bleeding
- Infection
- Urethral obstruction
- Urethral stricture
- Proctitis
- Rectal injury
- BOO

BILATERAL ORCHIECTOMY[5, 8, 18, 23, 32-33]
- Used for hormonal manipulation of metastatic disease
- Removes source of testicular androgen production

Procedure
- Local or general anesthesia
- Outpatient procedure
- Removal of both testicles through scrotal incision

Advantage
- Immediate reduction in testosterone levels
- Low cost, low morbidity
- No tumor flare
- Reduced bone pain
- No need for injections

Complications
- Infection and bleeding
- Hematoma

Pain Management
- Ice applications, scrotal support, oral analgesics, sitz baths when approved by urologist

Patient Education
- Wear scrotal support until pain is gone and wound has healed; perform wound care and watch for signs and symptoms of infection.
- Routine pre- and postoperative care
- Gauze fluff dressing
- Scrotal support
- Ice compresses
- Sitz baths when approved by urologist

Disadvantages
- Psychological effects
- Feelings of emasculation
- Side effects due to loss of testosterone (See Chapter 12 for hormonal therapy for management of side effects due to androgen ablative therapy.)

Complications (may be due to loss of testosterone)
- Loss of libido
- Impotency
- Hot flashes
- Osteoporosis
- Fatigue
- Loss of muscle mass

Psychosocial issues
- Scrotal prosthesis is available.
- Support group may be helpful with concerns over loss of manhood from procedure.

References
1. Held-Warmkessel J. Prostate cancer. In: Yarbro CH, Goodman M, Frogge MH, Groenwald SL, eds. *Cancer Nursing Principles and Practice.* 5th ed. Sudbury, Mass: Jones and Bartlett; 2000:1427–1451.
2. Klimaszewski AD, Karlowicz KA. Cancer of the male genitalia. In: Karlowicz KA, ed. *Urologic Nursing Principles and Practice.* Philadelphia, Pa: WB Saunders; 1995: 271–308.
3. Osborne DM. Surgical care of the patient with prostate cancer. In: Held-Warmkessel J, ed. *Contemporary Issues in Prostate Cancer: A Nursing Perspective.* Sudbury, Mass: Jones and Bartlett; 2000:117–134.
4. Berry DL. Bladder disturbances. In: Yarbro CH, Frogge MH, Goodman M, eds. C*ancer Symptom Management.* 3rd ed. Sudbury, Mass: Jones and Bartlett; 2004:493–504.
5. Held-Warmkessel J. Treatment of advanced prostate cancer. *Semin Oncol Nursing.* 2001;17:118–128.
6. Frydenberg M, Oesterling JE. Management of stage C (T3) prostate cancer: Nonradiation therapy. In: Raghavan D, Scher HI, Leibel SA, Lange PH, eds. *Principles and Practice of Genitourinary Oncology.* Philadelphia, Pa: Lippincott-Raven; 1997:535–541.
7. Moyad MA, Pienta KJ. *The ABC's of Advanced Prostate Cancer.* Chelsea, Mich: Sleeping Bear Press; 2000:55,88.
8. Klingman L. Interventions for male clients with reproductive problems. In: Ingatavicus DD, Workman ML, eds. *Medical-Surgical Nursing: Critical Thinking for Collaborative Care.* 4th ed. Philadelphia, Pa: WB Saunders; 2002:1782–1804.
9. Weaver J. Combating complications of transurethral surgery. *Nursing.* 2001;31:32hn1–2,32hn4.
10. Kilpatrick, JA. Urinary elimination. In: Potter PA, Perry AG, eds. *Fundamentals of Nursing.* 5th ed. Philadelphia, Pa: Mosby; 2001:1383–1435.
11. Ludwick, R. Urinary elimination. In: Perry AG, Potter PA, eds. *Clinical Nursing Skills & Techniques.* 5th ed. Philadelphia, Pa: Mosby; 2002:702–738.
12. Matassarin-Jacobs E. Nursing care of men with reproductive disorders. In: Black JM, Matassarin-Jacobs E, eds. *Medical-Surgical Nursing: Clinical Management for Continuity of Care.* 5th ed. Philadelphia, Pa: WB Saunders;1997:2343–2385.
13. Kirby RS, Christmas TJ, Brawer MK. *Prostate Cancer.* 2nd ed. London: Mosby; 2001:119–129,139–141,171–173.
14. National Comprehensive Cancer Network. Clinical Practice Guidelines in Oncology: Prostate Cancer 2004. Available at: http://www.nccn.org/professionals/physician _gls/PDF/prostate.pdf. Accessed June 22, 2004.

15. Goldenberg SL, Ramsey EW, Jewett MAS. Prostate cancer: 6. Surgical treatment of localized disease. *CMAJ.* 1998;159:1265–1271.
16. Pirtskhalaishvili G, Hrebinko RL, Nelson JB. The treatment of prostate cancer: an overview of current options. *Cancer Pract.* 2001;9:295–306.
17. Peschel RE, Colberg JW. Surgery, brachytherapy, and external-beam radiotherapy for early prostate cancer. *Lancet.* 2003;4:233–241.
18. Gray M. A prostate cancer primer. *Urol Nurs.* 2002;22:151–169.
19. Jani AB, Hellman S. Early prostate cancer: Clinical decision-making. (Prostate cancer III). *Lancet.* 2003;361:1045–1053.
20. Templeton H. The management of prostate cancer. *Nurs Stand.* 2003;17:45–55.
21. Marschke PS. The role of surgery in the treatment of prostate cancer. *Semin Oncol Nurs.* 2001;17:85–89.
22. Sokoloff MH, Brendler CB. Indications and contraindications for nerve-sparing radical prostatectomy. *Urol Clin North Am.* 2001;28:535–544.
23. National Cancer Institute. Prostate cancer (PDQ): Treatment health professional version. Available at: http://cancernet.nci.nih.gov/cancertopics/pdq/treatment/prostate/healthprofessional. Accessed June 22, 2004.
24. Ellsworth P, Heaney J, Gill C. *100 Questions & Answers About Prostate Cancer.* Sudbury, Mass; Jones and Bartlett; 2003:157.
25. Karius DL, O'Brien SM, Dumas MC. Oncology nursing practice. In: Volgezang NJ, Scardino PT, Shipley WU, Coffey DS, eds. *Comprehensive Textbook of Genitourinary Oncology.* 2nd ed. Philadelphia, Pa: Lippincott Williams & Wilkins; 2000:49–55.
26. Held-Warmkessel J. What your patient needs to know about prostate cancer. *Nursing.* 2002;32:36–43.
27. Schmidt JD, Doyle J, Larison S. Prostate cryoablation: Update 1998. *CA Cancer J Clin.* 1998;48:239–253.
28. Bermejo CE, Plisters LL. Cryotherapy for prostate cancer. *Expert Rev Anticancer Ther.* 2003;3:393–401.
29. Moul JW. Treatment options for prostate cancer: Part 2–early and late stage and hormone refractory disease. *Am J Manag Care.* 1998;4:1171–1182.
30. Shinohara K. Prostate cancer: cryotherapy. *Urol Clin North Am.* 2003;30:725–736.
31. Leininger SM. Managing patients with cryosurgical ablation of the prostate and liver. *Medsurg Nurs.* 1997;6:359–363,386.
32. Gleave ME, Bruchovsky N, Moore MJ, Venner P. Prostate cancer: 9. Treatment of advanced disease. *CMAJ.* 1999;160:225–232.
33. McLeod DG, Vogelzang NJ. Initial management of metastatic prostate cancer. In: Vogelzang NJ, Scardino PT, Shipley WU, Coffey DS, eds. *Comprehensive Textbook of Genitourinary Oncology.* 2nd ed. Philadelphia, Pa: Lippincott Williams & Wilkins, 2000:824–841.

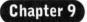

Laparoscopic Radical Prostatectomy

INTRODUCTION
- Type of minimally invasive surgery

CANDIDATE SELECTION[1, 2]
- No major medical problems such as cardiac or pulmonary disease
- PSA < 15 ng/mL
- Localized disease
- Moderately to well-differentiated cells on pathology
- Life expectancy of 15 years or more
- No prior pelvic radiation therapy
- Not obese
- No multiple abdominal or pelvic surgical or other procedures

PREOPERATIVE CARE
- Surgeon-provided patient education includes
  - Procedure
  - Risks and benefits
  - Alternative modalities of cancer treatment
- Common risks
  - Infection
  - Bleeding, need for blood transfusions
  - Erectile dysfunction, impotence
  - Urinary incontinence
  - Anesthesia complications
  - Need to convert to open prostatectomy during laparoscopic approach

Preoperative Tests
- Complete blood count (CBC)
- Chemistry panel
- PSA
- EKG
- Chest X-ray
- Type and screen or cross-match

Preadmission Patient Education and Assessment
- Performed in person or by phone
- Includes the following
  - Past medical and surgical history
  - Past and current medications including over-the-counter medications, herbal, and other dietary supplements
  - Allergies

- Herbal medications are to be discontinued 7–10 days before surgery.
- Anticoagulants are usually discontinued 7 days before surgery.
- Dependent on the patient's history, cardiac and antihypertensive medications are taken the morning of surgery.
- Postdischarge needs assessment is performed.
- Patient's understanding of surgical procedure
- Bowel prep instructions, oral and written
- Day of surgery instructions include NPO, arrival time, surgical preparation, amount of time needed for preparation, time in OR, PACU, and hospitalization processes.
- Pain management—IV, oral, PCA pump use and precautions
- Time for patient questions

Preoperative Care

- Similar to the care provided for open prostatectomy, general abdominal surgery, general anesthesia
- Patient education—pain management, postoperative care
- Vital signs, pulse oximetry
- Skin assessment
- Medical and surgical conditions that would be affected by intraoperative positioning
- Removal of removable metal objects
- IV fluids, prophylactic antibiotics
- DVT prophylaxis—elastic stockings
- Patient warming blanket

INTRAOPERATIVE CARE[3]

- Patient identification
- Careful patient positioning—supine, low lithotomy, Trendelenburg—to enhance access to patient for procedure and avoid cardiac and pulmonary compromise and stress, and stress on joints, nerves, and blood vessels
- Sequential compression stockings
- Safety and securement to OR table
- Patient warming
- Skin preparation from xyphoid process to upper thigh including genitals and perineal area using antimicrobial skin prep solution
- Indwelling urinary catheter inserted into bladder
- Time out
- Equipment set up and check
- Needle and sponge counts
- Procedural approaches[4–6]
  - Transperitoneal—abdominal cavity insufflated with carbon dioxide. Trocars are inserted via small incisions. Periprostatic and prostatic tissue removed and the urethra anastomosed. Indwelling urethral catheter is placed to check the anastomosis for leaking.
  - Extraperitoneal—Similar procedure with less risk of bowel injury. Trendelenburg positioning not as extreme. Procedure done via retropubic space. Less risk of damage to intraperitoneal structures. Shorter operative time. Approach similar to traditional radical prostatectomy.
- Outcomes are similar for both approaches in terms of positive margins, potency rates, and continence rates.

Robotics

- Provides surgical assistance by improving surgical dexterity lost with the use of laparoscopic equipment.
- Heavy, expensive, and time consuming to use
- Requires larger operating room

POSTOPERATIVE CARE

- See **Table 9–1** and **Table 9–2**.
- Routine PACU care and then surgical floor care
- Indwelling urinary catheter is to gravity and is not to be manipulated or irrigated, which could damage the urethral anastomosis. If there are catheter problems, the urologist is to be notified.
- Sequential compression stockings and ambulation on postop day 1

TABLE 9–1 Sample Postoperative Orders for Laparoscopic Radical Prostatectomy

1. Transfer to PACU–surgical floor
2. S/P laparoscopic radical prostatectomy
3. Condition stable
4. Diet: NPO except ice chips; not to exceed 30 ml /hr.
5. Activity: Bedrest tonight then OOB TID in a.m. Progressive ambulation as tolerated.
6. Vital signs per PACU then every 2 hours times 2, then every 4 hours if vital signs stable.
7. Strict intake & output
8. IV fluids: Present IV @ 125 mL per hour then D5-1/2 NS @ 125 mL per hour.
9. Labs: CBC, Basic Metabolic Panel in PACU and repeat in a.m.
10. Meds: Cefazolin 1 gram IVPB every 8 hours for 24 hours

    Morphine sulfate 2 mg IV every 2 hours prn mild pain, and 3 mg IV every 2 hours moderate pain

    Acetaminophen 650 mg PO every 4 hours prn for headaches or temperature greater than 100.4° F

    Oxybutynin 5 mg PO every 8 hours prn bladder spasms
11. Respiratory: O2 @ 2 liters per minute per nasal cannula
12. Sequential compression stocking device
13. Indwelling urinary catheter to gravity. DO NOT manipulate catheter.
14. Drain to suction bulb.
15. Call MD if: Temp ≥ 101° F; pulse less than 50 or greater than 130; systolic BP less than 90 or greater than 180; diastolic BP greater than 90; urine output less than 240 mL/8 hour period.

PACU, postanesthesia care unit; O2, oxygen; prn, as needed; BP, blood pressure; IV, intravenous; CBC, complete blood count; D5-1/2 NS, 5% dextrose in 1/2 normal saline; NPO, nothing by mouth; OOB, out of bed; TID, 3 times a day; S/P, status post.
Source: Bickert D. Laparoscopic radical prostatectomy. In: Held-Warmkessel, J., ed. *Contemporary Issues in Prostate Cancer: A Nursing Perspective* (2nd ed). Jones and Bartlett Publishers, 2006, 183–201. Reprinted with permission by Jones and Bartlett Publishers.

TABLE 9-2 Nursing Care Plan Laparoscopic Radical Prostatectomy

	Nursing Diagnosis	Expected Outcome	Nursing Interventions
Preoperative	1. Risk of anxiety due to knowledge deficit	The patient demonstrates understanding of the procedure including risks and benefits. The patient participates in the decision regarding his care.	1. Assess the patient's level of understanding and readiness to learn. 2. Assess support available to patient. 3. Assess that patient understands upcoming procedure as explained by surgeon, and if necessary, coordinate further follow-up with surgeon. 4. Explain procedures to be carried out such as preoperative preparation, pain scale, and pain control. 5. Allow time for patient and support person to ask questions. 6. Evaluate patient's understanding.
	2. Risk of anxiety due to altered physical state (potential for urinary incontinence and/or erectile dysfunction)	The patient expresses understanding of possible physical alterations.	1. Allow patient to verbalize concerns or feelings. 2. Involve support person as possible. 3. Provide emotional support for patient.
	3. Risk of hypothermia	Patient's temperature remains within normal limits throughout the perioperative period.	1. Apply warming blanket in the preoperative area, reapply immediately after positioning, and in the PACU. 2. Utilize fluid warmer for IV fluids intraoperatively.
Intraoperative	1. Risk of injury due to inadequate preoperative preparation	Patient is free from injury.	1. Confirm NPO status. 2. Confirm known allergies.

continues

TABLE 9–2 Nursing Care Plan Laparoscopic Radical Prostatectomy, continued

Nursing Diagnosis	Expected Outcome	Nursing Interventions
Intraoperative, cont'd		3. Patient identity and procedure to be performed is confirmed with patient, surgical schedule, history, physical, and consent. A time-out is performed by the operating room team before the start of the procedure to again confirm correct patient, site, and procedure.
2. Risk of injury to skin, musculoskeletal, and/or neurological systems from positioning	Patient is free from signs or symptoms of injury related to positioning.	1. Assess patient for any skin or musculoskeletal issues or conditions that would be impacted or exacerbated by routine positioning. 2. Utilize protective devices and padding to position the patient and maintain body alignment.
3. Risk of injury to skin from pooling of prep solutions and/or improper placement of electrosurgical grounding pad	Patient is free from skin damage, including redness, blisters, and burns.	1. Assess patient for allergies to prep solutions. 2. Place towels along edges of surgical prep site to prevent pooling of prep solution under patient. 3. Place grounding pad on anterior thigh or other nonbony prominence area.
4. Risk of impaired gas exchange from positioning	The patient's pulmonary function is consistent with baseline levels.	1. Assist anesthesiologist as needed with induction and intubation. 2. Assess patient for adequate chest expansion after positioning.

continues

TABLE 9–2 Nursing Care Plan Laparoscopic Radical Prostatectomy, continued

	Nursing Diagnosis	Expected Outcome	Nursing Interventions
Intraoperative, cont'd	5. Risk of infection	The patient is free from signs or symptoms of infection.	1. Infuse prophylactic antibiotics as ordered within one hour of incision time. 2. Perform skin prep per surgeon preference. 3. Monitor and maintain body temperature utilizing warming blanket, warmed fluids, and limiting skin exposure. 4. Monitor and maintain sterile technique throughout the procedure.
	6. Risk of retained foreign objects due to surgical procedure	The patient is free from foreign objects. All sponge and needle counts are correct prior to the patient's discharge from the operating room.	1. Needle, sponge, and instrument counts are performed prior to the start of the case. 2. All items added during the case will be counted and documented. 3. Counts will be conducted at the end of the case per protocol.
	7. Risk of loss of privacy and dignity due to physical exposure	The patient's dignity will be maintained throughout the surgical procedure.	1. Keep operating room doors closed and limit personnel in room to those necessary for the case. 2. Obtain patient's permission preoperatively for any observers to surgical procedure.
Postoperative	1. Risk of cardiopulmonary compromise	Patient's cardiac and respiratory status is consistent with baseline level.	1. Monitor vital signs closely including temperature, blood pressure, heart rate, respiratory rate, and quality and pulse oximetry readings.

continues

TABLE 9–2 Nursing Care Plan Laparoscopic Radical Prostatectomy, continued

Nursing Diagnosis	Expected Outcome	Nursing Interventions
Postoperative cont'd		2. Administer oxygen, fluids and/or blood products as prescribed by surgeon or anesthesia provider. 3. Monitor intake and output q4 hours. 4. Notify physician of any abnormal laboratory results. 5. Monitor for signs and symptoms of deep vein thrombosis.
2. Risk of inadequate pain management	Patient will meet self-determined pain goal.	1. Assess patient's reported pain based on a 1–10 pain scale. 2. Assess patient for nonverbal clues to comfort level including changes in vital signs, nonverbal facial expressions, or restless behavior. 3. Medicate patient per orders as needed for pain. 4. Reassess pain level at appropriate interval after pain medication.
3. Risk of gastrointestinal compromise	Patient will have normal gastrointestinal function.	1. Maintain NPO status and advance diet per physician orders. 2. Monitor intake and output q4 hours.

continues

TABLE 9–2 Nursing Care Plan Laparoscopic Radical Prostatectomy, continued

	Nursing Diagnosis	Expected Outcome	Nursing Interventions
Postoperative, cont'd	4. Risk of knowledge deficit for postdischarge care including pain management, wound care, and foley catheter care	Patient will verbalize understanding of pain management and wound and urinary catheter care.	1. Instruct patient and support person regarding pain control including pain medication and alternative nonpharmacologic techniques. 2. Instruct patient and support person regarding wound and indwelling urinary catheter care. 3. Ask patient to redemonstrate wound and catheter care. 4. Allow time for patient and support person to ask questions. 5. Provide patient with written instructions for reference at home.

Source: Bickert D. Laproscopic radial prostatectomy. In: Held-Warmkessel, J., ed. *Contemporary Issues in Prostate Cancer: A Nursing Perspective* (2nd ed). Jones and Bartlett Publishers, 2006, 183–201. Reprinted with permission by Jones and Bartlett Publishers

TABLE 9–3 Laparoscopic Prostatectomy Sample Perioperative Data

Author	Number of Patients	Procedure Performed	Operative Time	Conversion to Open Procedure (%)	Transfusion Rate (%)
Guillonneau & Vallacien[10]	350	LRP (Transperitoneal)	217 minutes	7	5.7
Hoznek et al.[11]	200	LRP (Transperitoneal)	210 minutes (does not include first 20 cases)	0	3
Rassweiler et al.[12]	100	LRP (Transperitoneal)	278 minutes	5	31
Turk et al.[13]	125	LRP (Transperitoneal)	287	2	9
Bollens et al.[14]	85	LRP (Extraperitoneal)	255	0	2
Stolzenburg et al.[8]	300	LRP (Extraperitoneal)	150	0	1.3
Hoznek et al.[15]	20	LRP (Extraperitoneal)	Not available	0	10

Source: Bickert D. Laproscopic radial prostatectomy. In: Held-Warmkessel, J., ed. *Contemporary Issues in Prostate Cancer: A Nursing Perspective* (2nd ed). Jones and Bartlett Publishers, 2006, 183–201. Reprinted with permission by Jones and Bartlett Publishers.

- Antibiotics
- Pain medications
- Length of stay—approximately 2 days
- Strict I&O
- Respiratory—coughing and deep breathing
- Nursing assessment of GI, respiratory, cardiovascular, urinary tract, wound, drain(s), catheter, and pain
- Monitor for postoperative complications such as infection, bleeding, DVT, pulmonary embolus, or dislodgement of indwelling urinary catheter.
- Patient education—wound care, signs and symptoms of infection, care of indwelling urinary catheter, ambulation, restrictions, monitoring for and reporting to urologist the presence of clots, blood, odor, or cloudiness in urine

OUTCOMES[8-15]

- See **Table 9–3**.
- Possible complications include intraoperative injury to bowel, ureters, and urine leaking from anastomosis into abdominal cavity.
- Long operative times increase risk of complications
- Shorter length of stay
- Catheter remains in place 4–10 days, dependent on urologist preference
- Cancer control
  - Positive margins—9–26%[8]
  - Continence rates—81–95%[8]
  - Impotency rates—50–70%[8-15]

I thank Denise Bickert, MS, RN, CNOR, for her review of this chapter.

References

1. Cathelineau X, Arroyo C, Rozet F, et al. Laparoscopic radical prostatectomy: the new gold standard? *Current Urology Reports.* 2004;5:108–114.
2. Steinber A, Gill I. Laparoscopic prostatectomy: a promising option on the treatment of prostate cancer. *Cleveland Clin J Med.* 2004;71:113–121.
3. Meeker M, Rothrock J. *Alexander's Care of the Patient in Surgery.* 11th ed. St Louis, Mo: Mosby; 1999:509.
4. Guillonneau B, Rozet F, Barret E, et al. Advanced urologic laparoscopy: laparoscopic radical prostatectomy: assessment after 240 procedures. *Urol Clin North Am.* 2001;28:189–202.
5. Stolzenburg J, Truss M, Bekos A, et al. Does the extraperitoneal laparoscopic approach improve the outcome of radical prostatectomy? *Curr Urol Rep.* 2004;5:115–122.
6. Bollens R, Roumeguere T, Schulman C. Extraperitoneal laparoscopic RP: the Brussels technique. *Contemp Urol Arch.* August 2004;16:13–22.
7. Lanfranco A, Castellanos A, Desai J, et al. Robotic surgery: a current perspective. *Ann Surg.* 2004;239:14–21.
8. Bollens R, Roumeguere T, Bossche M, et al. Comparison of laparoscopic radical prostatectomy techniques. *Curr Urol Rep.* 2002;3:148–151.
9. Bickert D, Frickel D. Laparoscopic prostatectomy. *AORN J.* 2002;75:760–788.
10. Guillonneau B, Cathelineau X, Doublet JD, et al. Laparoscopic prostatectomy: the lessons learned. *J Endourol.* 2001;15:441–445.

11. Hoznek A, Salomon L, Olsson LE, et al. Laparoscopic radical prostatectomy: the Creteil experience. *Eur Urol.* 2001;40:38–45.
12. Rassweiler J, Sentker L, Seeman O. et al. Heilbronn laparoscopic radical prostatectomy. technique and results after 100 cases. *Eur Urol.* 2001;40:54–64.
13. Turk I, Deger S, Winkelmann B, et al. Laparoscopic radical prostatectomy: technical aspects and experience with 125 cases. *Eur Urol.* 2001;40:46–53.
14. Bollens R, Vanden Bossche M, Roumeguere T, et al. Extraperitoneal laparoscopic prostatectomy. Results after 50 cases. *Eur Urol.* 2001;40:65–69.
15. Hoznek A, Antiphon P, Borkowski T, et al. Assessment of surgical technique and perioperative morbidity associated with extraperitoneal versus transperitoneal laparoscopic radical prostatectomy. *Urology.* 2003;61:617–622.

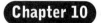

External Beam Radiation Therapy

INTRODUCTION[1-6]

- Use of ionizing radiation to damage or break cellular DNA strands
- DNA damage may affect single-stands or double-strands of DNA. Double-strand damage is lethal to cells, but cells may not die until they try to reproduce.
- Prostate cancer has a slow rate of growth, and cells may not attempt cellular reproduction until after the treatments are completed.
- Treatments are administered 5 days per week over a predetermined period of time and a specific amount of radiation is given every day.
- The radiation dose is measured in Gray (Gy) and delivered in a daily dose called a fraction. 1.8–2.0 Gy are typically administered each treatment day.
- Damage to normal body tissues causes the side effects seen with radiation therapy. The body is able to repair many of the tissue injuries with cellular reproduction.
- Outcome comparison between radical prostatectomy and radiation therapy is not easy as there are no prospective randomized trials comparing the two approaches. For early prostate cancer, 10-year survival rates are similar between radiation therapy and radical prostatectomy.
- Radiation therapy is often recommended for the older patient (> 70) with a higher grade tumor and poorer health.
- For T3–T4 tumors, radiation therapy with or without hormonal therapy is usually recommended.

PRETREATMENT WORKUP

Tissue diagnosis required to confirm diagnosis
- Transrectal ultrasound (TRUS)-guided biopsy
- Transurethral resection of the prostate (TURP) (incidental finding)

Workup includes
- Detailed clinical history
- General physical assessment
- Digital rectal examination (DRE)

Other studies may include
- Computed tomography (CT) scan or magnetic resonance imaging (MRI) of the abdomen and pelvis
- Radioisotope total body bone scan
- Chest radiography
- Ultrasound of the kidneys and bladder
- Some tests, such as CT and bone scan, may not be done due to low risk of metastatic disease.
- Cystoscopy

Laboratory tests
- Current PSA level and all other available past PSA levels, if available

Other lab tests
- Complete blood cell count
- Urine analysis
- Serum chemistry panel
- Baseline liver function and testosterone levels

SIMULATION/TREATMENT PLANNING BASED ON RADIATION TREATMENT SELECTION

Treatment Options/Choices
- Three-dimensional conformal radiation therapy (3D CRT)—Available due to advances in computer and software technology. Multiple beams of radiation delivered to tumor in a more precise manner. Higher dose to prostate is possible due to better target confirmation while reducing the volume of normal tissue in radiation treatment field. Goal is fewer radiation-related bowel and bladder side effects.
- IMRT—Radiation is planned using computer-generated algorithm so that beams deliver radiation to a more precisely targeted area of the prostate and surrounding tissue while sparing normal tissue beyond the capability of 3-D CRT. Organs to be avoided include bowel, bladder, femoral heads, and bulb of penis.
- Image-Guided RT—A method of using images to accurately target the daily tumor location with respect to changes in body position and internal organ movement.

Treatment Planning Process/Simulation Procedure
- Registered radiation therapist and radiation oncologist perform simulation.
- During treatment planning, equipment simulates actual treatment and simulation is required prior to initiating treatment
- Dedicated X-ray, CT scanner, or MRI may be used to perform simulation.
- Used to determine beam arrangements, couch-gantry position, beam geometry
- For X-ray machines, fluoroscopy is used to outline radiation field borders and chose the center of the treatment beam.
- Contrast dye may be instilled into bladder and/or rectum for better visualization of these tissues.
- A urethrogram may be done to better define the prostate apex.
- Procedure performed on narrow table and takes at least 1 hour.
- Skin markings (tattoos) placed—Temporary or permanent (temporary marks must not be removed) after radiation oncologist has defined target.
- Individually fabricated, rigid immobilization device (alpha cradle or thermoplastics) may be made to allow for delivery of radiation to same area each day by promoting proper positioning of the patient on the table each day. Proper positioning is crucial for daily treatments in order to ensure that the target is in the radiation beam.

EXTERNAL BEAM RADIATION THERAPY

Introduction
- Also called teletherapy, radiotherapy, irradiation
- Variety of radiation-producing equipment available
- Deliver different energy levels; deliver to different tissue depths

Treatment Volume/Technique

- Radiation delivered using several beams—typically anterioposterior (AP/PA) and laterally opposed. IMRT uses 5–9 treatment fields.
- Administered daily, five times a week (Monday to Friday most typically)
- Daily dose is 1.8–2.0 Gy.
- Verification films are taken weekly to ensure accurate delivery of the radiation treatment to the target area.
- Size of radiation portal differs for each patient—includes prostate gland and occasionally the seminal vesicles and pelvic lymph nodes.
- Lymph modes may be included in the treatment field, typically for patients with intermediate- or high-risk disease. If they are treated, a dose of 45–50 Gy is typically administered.
- Patients at high risk may receive whole pelvic radiation therapy plus a prostate boost—a formula and/or a table is used to determine risk of lymph node metastases.

Stage T1–T2

- May be treated with external beam radiation therapy, but these patients also have other treatment options such as surgery or brachytherapy.

Stages T3–T4

- Usually treated with external beam radiation therapy *with or without* hormonal therapy

Metastatic Disease/Palliative Interventions[7–9]

- Treatment of painful bone metastases
  - Single or multiple treatments may be used.
  - 8 Gy in one fraction, 20 Gy in 4–5 fractions, or 30 Gy in 10 fractions
- Treatment to reduce obstructive urinary symptoms
- Spinal cord compression requires emergency treatment.
  - Dexamethasone
  - Total dose 30–40 Gy
  - Surgery may also be indicated.
- Manage bleeding

Postprostatectomy Treatment[8–11]

- Absolute and relative indications for treatment include patients with positive surgical margins, seminal vesicle involvement, detectable PSA postoperatively, local disease recurrence, Gleason score ≥ 7, and pathologic T3 and T4 tumors.
- PSA levels after prostatectomy with removal of all malignant and normal cells should be at undetectable levels. For patients with rising PSA levels, disease may be local or micrometastatic. Additional treatment may be appropriate with 45–70 Gy administered to the tumor bed. Hormonal therapy may be administered to potentially reduce the rate of freedom from PSA failure.
- PSA levels after radiation therapy—Level not well defined due to presence of residual viable prostate cells producing PSA; serial rising PSA is a more effective indicator of biochemical failure.

Total Androgen Suppression

- May improve local control, reduce tumor volume (see Chapter 12)

THREE-DIMENSIONAL CONFORMAL RADIATION THERAPY[12-13]

Introduction

- Made possible by newer computers and software
- Higher radiation dose delivery to tumor and reduced delivery to normal structures
- Borders of treatment field are more clearly defined.
- Doses of radiation delivered are limited by the normal surrounding structures—bowel and bladder.
- Less rectal toxicity even though higher doses of radiation are administered

Three-Dimensional (3D) Planning

- Use of CT images to create a 3D view of the prostate and surrounding tissues
- Simulation performed as previously described
- Simulation and 3D films used to plan treatment
- Immobilization cast often made to aid in daily delivery of treatment so that radiation is accurately administered to the treatment field
- Doses researched in clinical trials ranged between 68.4 Gy and 79.2 GY and are under evaluation and were well tolerated.

EXTERNAL BEAM SIDE EFFECTS

- Acute side effects develop during or up to 90 days after completion of radiation therapy.
- Late side effects develop > 90 days after completion of radiation therapy.
- Severity related to radiation dose (total and fraction), volume, type (photon versus proton), and site of treatment and patient tolerance
- IMRT causes fewer side effects because of tight beam distribution and radiation delivery.

Bowel[14-17]

Acute toxicity

- More common when the abdomen or pelvis is irradiated
- Inflammation of bowel and/or rectal mucosa develops.
- Related to dose and volume of bowel/rectum in treatment field
- Begins after 15–30 Gy has been administered (week 2–3 of treatment), may be delayed with IMRT
- Symptoms include
  - Diarrhea (ranges from mild to severe)
  - Abdominal cramps
  - Tenesmus
  - Proctalgia
  - Rectal bleeding
- Rectal bleeding may be exacerbated by presence of preexisting hemorrhoids.
- Diarrhea may result in dehydration and electrolyte imbalance
- Managed with antidiarrheal medications (see **Table 10–1**)
- Nursing assessment
  - Amount, consistency, and frequency of diarrhea
  - Rectal skin integrity
  - Fluid balance—presence of dehydration: assess for dry oral mucosa, poor skin turgor, and determination of fluid intake past 24 hours; assess color and volume of urine output and volume of liquid stool.

TABLE 10-1 Antidiarrheal Agents

Drug	Dose	Frequency	Partial List of Potential Side Effects	Contraindications	Patient Education
Diphenoxylate hydrochloride with atropine sulfate	5 mg for initial control, then reduce to meet individual needs; control may be maintained with 5 mg daily	2 tablets qid	Paresthesia, lethargy, sedation, drowsiness, restlessness, headache, paralytic ileus, vomiting, nausea, anorexia, abdominal discomfort, urinary retention, flushing, dryness of skin and mucous membranes, blurred vision, rash	Hypersensitivity, obstructive jaundice, cirrhosis, pseudomembranous enterocolitis, MAO inhibitors	Increase fluid intake to at least 3000 mL/day. Keep record of frequency of bowel movements and be alert for constipation. Report if diarrhea does not improve after a few days, if blood is noted in stool, or if fever is present.
Loperamide	2 mg (5 mL/tsp)	4 tsp or 2 capsules after first loose bowel movement, then 2 tsp or 1 capsule after each subsequent loose bowel movement	Abdominal pain, distention, or discomfort; nausea, vomiting, constipation, drowsiness or dizziness, dry mouth, rash	History of liver disease, pseudomembranous colitis	Patients instructed to report any of the following symptoms: muscle weakness, anorexia, vomiting, drowsiness, irritability.
Paregoric	0.3–1 mL; mix with sufficient water to ensure passage to the stomach	qd–qid	Nausea, vomiting, physical dependency with long-term use, dizziness, lightheadedness	None significant	
Kaolin-pectin	60–120 mL	After each loose bowel movement	None significant	Suspected obstructive bowel lesions; may reduce absorption of other PO drugs	

qid, four times daily; qd, every day; MAOIs, monoamine oxidase inhibitors; PO, oral.
Data compiled from Wilkes[17] and Nursing 2005 Drug Handbook[16]

Source: Volpe H, Watkins SV. Radiation Therapy. In: Held-Warmkessel, J., ed. *Contemporary Issues in Prostate Cancer: A Nursing Perspective* (2nd ed). Jones and Bartlett Publishers, 2006, 202–228. Reprinted with permission by Jones and Bartlett Publishers.

- Patient education
  - Use of antidiarrheal medications (see **Table 10–1**)
  - Low-residue diet (see **Table 10–2**)
  - Increased fluid intake
  - Increased intake of electrolyte-rich liquids and foods
  - Sitz baths for proctitis, rectal discomfort, and hemorrhoids
  - Use of prescribed hydrocortisone-based medication or anti-inflammatory suppositories

Late toxicity: 1–3% of patients
- Persistent bowel changes produce symptoms of
  - Diarrhea
  - Fistula formation
  - Perforation
  - Bleeding due to incomplete or delayed bowel mucosa healing, edema, fibrosis, or vascular insufficiency
  - Chronic bowel changes—edema, fibrosis, poor blood supply
- Chronic intermittent bleeding—treatment with laser or fulguration
- Intestinal obstruction
- Often requires gastroenterology consult

Skin[18]

- Dose-dependent radiation reaction
- Thin skin in area at greater risk of altered integrity
- Radiation produces epidermal and dermal cell loss and damage to endothelial microvasculature.
- Perineal or intergluteal areas affected
- Reaction includes erythema, pain, and dry or moist desquamation.
- Caused by inflammation, cell loss, and serosanguineous drainage
- Produces pain/discomfort
- Nursing assessment—altered skin integrity, monitor for infection
- Patient education
  - Good perineal hygiene—wash perineal area with tepid water and pat dry
  - Avoid soap, powders, lotions, creams, and other topical agents applied to skin unless prescribed by radiation oncologist.
  - Use sitz baths.
  - Wear cotton undergarments and loose clothing.
  - Correctly use and apply prescribed skin treatments.
  - Avoid oil-based skin preparations.
  - Use water-based skin emulsions.

Urinary Tract (Cystitis)[2, 19, 20]

- Common acute side effect
- Etiology not well understood
  - Irritation, edema, inflammation and vascular changes to urothelium, muscle, and blood vessels
  - Reduced bladder capacity due to vascular damage and collagen deposits
  - Cause irritative voiding symptoms
- Assess patients for urinary tract infections and send urine specimen for culture.
- Acute symptoms begin weeks 3–5 of treatment and resolve 2–8 weeks after completion of radiation therapy.
  - Dysuria
  - Frequency due to irritative symptoms and reduced bladder capacity

TABLE 10–2 Diarrhea

What can cause diarrhea?

Cancer treatment, drugs, or infection can cause diarrhea. When this happens a change in diet or medicine may help. Your doctor may order some tests to find out the cause.

What can I take to stop diarrhea?

Imodium is one medicine that your doctor may order for you. Follow your doctor's orders on how to take it. They may be different than package instructions.

How can food affect diarrhea?

Certain parts of food may have an effect on diarrhea. Fiber (roughage) found in whole grains, breads, cereal, raw fruit, and vegetables with skin or seeds can make diarrhea worse.

Milk or milk products can cause or worsen diarrhea. These foods contain the sugar lactose. If your digestive system does not break down lactose, you may have cramping, gas, or diarrhea. Low-lactose dairy products or substitutes such as soybean milk and ice cream may help. Your doctor may also suggest that you take enzyme pills before eating regular dairy products.

Foods that are very high in fat may also make diarrhea worse and should be avoided.

The fluids lost during diarrhea must be replaced, but all fluids are not equal when it comes to replacing fluid losses. Alcohol and drinks with caffeine (such as coffee, cola, and strong tea) should be limited as they may actually increase fluid loss. Apricot, peach, or pear nectar and fruit-ades are good choices for fluid replacement. Take liquids between meals instead of with them.

Along with fluids, potassium can be lost and needs to be replaced. Below is a list of foods high in potassium, which you may be able to tolerate. Potassium pills may also be ordered by your doctor.

Food high in potassium

- Apricots (canned and nectar)
- Bananas
- Orange juice
- Pineapple juice
- Peach nectar
- Tomato (juice, soup, V-8)
- Carrot (juice and canned)
- Potato (white or sweet)
- Squash (winter, acorn, butternut)
- Spinach
- Beef, fish
- Milk, Lactaid, soy milk

Call your doctor if you have:

- Diarrhea more than 4 times a day
- Temperature of 100.5°F or higher
- A hard, distended abdomen (belly)
- Abdominal pain

Eating tips if you have diarrhea

Suggest	Avoid
Low-lactose milk and milk products (for example, Lactaid)	Regular milk, cream, half & half milk products, and cheese
Aged cheese (such as cheddar)	Legumes, nuts, seeds
Yogurt	Fried meat, chicken, fish, and eggs
Soybean milk products (Nursoy, Soyalac, Tofutti)	Whole grains: bran, brown rice, whole wheat bread, whole wheat pasta, whole wheat crackers, and high-fiber cereal

continues

TABLE 10-2 Diarrhea, continued

Eating tips if you have diarrhea

Suggest	Avoid
Nutrition supplements (Ensure, Resource Fruit Beverages, Enlive, Biocare Drink Mix)	Prunes and prune juice
	Potato skin
	Raw fruit and vegetables
	Dried fruit
Baked/boiled/stewed meat, fish and chicken	Fried snack food
Eggs	Gravy (large amounts)
Refined grains and cereals: white bread and rice, cream of wheat or cream of rice, and noodles or pasta	Drinks with caffeine
All cooked vegetables (especially carrots, beets, and mashed potatoes).	Popcorn
Canned fruit and applesauce	
Juice and nectars	
Bananas	
Nondairy creamer	
Margarine	
Gatorade	

The examples used may not be available at all stores. Ask your doctor, dietitian, or nurse for other tips if needed.

Source: Courtesy of Fox Chase Cancer Center. Used with permission.

- Hesitancy
- Urgency
- Hematuria in part due to vascular changes of the bladder

Acute cystitis treatment
- Managed with medications such as
    1. Urinary anesthetics: phenazopyridine hydrochloride or smooth muscle anti-spasmodics such as flavoxate hydrochloride, hyoscyamine sulfate, oxybutynin chloride
        - Assess patient for central nervous system stimulation.
        - Cardiac side effects include palpitations, hypertension, arrhythmias.
        - Educate patient to report side effects.
    2. Alpha-1 blocker therapy: terazocin, doxazosin mesylate, tamsulosin hydrochloride
        - Assess patient for hypotension.
        - Educate patient to report signs and symptoms of hypotension.
- Nursing assessment
    - Assess impact of altered urinary elimination on patient's quality of life.
    - Monitor for changes in blood pressure when patient is prescribed α-1 blockers or antispasmodic medications.
    - Monitor patient for other drug-related side effects.

- Patient education
  - Increase fluid intake to 2 liters/day, unless contraindicated by preexisting medical conditions.
  - Use of prescribed medication and drug side effect profile
  - Avoid bladder-irritating substances: alcohol, caffeine, tobacco, and spices.
- Chronic toxicity
  - Hematuria from mucosal inflammation or telangiectasia
  - Cystoscopy is a useful diagnostic and therapeutic procedure.
  - Must rule out urinary tract infection.
- Rare side effects—incontinence, urethral stricture

Sexual Functioning[2, 21]

- Erectile dysfunction is caused by radiation-induced injury to blood vessels and nerves that are involved with erectile function and/or by direct damage to the penile bulb or crura of the penis.
- Preexisting medical problems, psychological factors, and age also influence erectile function.
- Changes may not occur until a year or more after radiation therapy.
- Younger men are more likely to remain potent.
- Nursing assessment of sexual issues and concerns begins prior to starting radiation therapy.
- Interventions include education and appropriate referrals.

Fatigue[22–23]

- Common acute radiation side effect, usually mild to moderate in severity
- Begins around week 4 and lasts for about 1 month after treatment completed
- May be caused by multiple factors including anemia, pain, diarrhea, tumor degradation, hormonal therapy, and transportation requirements for daily treatment
- Nursing assessment
  - Severity of fatigue, causes, and impact on quality of life
- Patient education
  - Energy conservation techniques, rest
  - Use of available resources

Myelosuppression[14, 23–24]

- Forty percent of bone marrow is located in pelvis, but myelosuppression is rare with radiation therapy alone.
- Radiation to a large field increases risk. Other risk factors include metastatic disease and older age.
- Incidence of treatment interruptions for myelosuppression is rare.
- Does not usually require treatment. Hemoglobin drop is usually < 0.5g/dL unless patient is receiving combined modality radiation therapy and hormonal therapy, which may cause decreased hemoglobin levels of up to 4 g/dL.
- Nursing assessment
  - Assess for presence of infection, bleeding, fatigue, dyspnea, dyspnea on exertion, headache, chest pain, paresthesias, or other signs and symptoms of anemia.
  - Monitor complete blood count results.
- Patient education regarding signs and symptoms of myelosuppression and self-care measures

COMBINATION THERAPY[25-28]

Introduction

- Hormonal therapy is used before, during, or after definitive radiation therapy to improve outcome.
- Enhances synergy between the modalities
- Used in patients with locally or regionally advanced disease
- Used in patients with moderate- to high-grade cancer
- Used with large tumors to reduce tumor size when given prior to radiation therapy
- Reduces risk of local failure by almost half and PSA failure by a factor of 2.5 in some instances.[26]
- Combination therapy may increase diarrhea.
- Additional hormone-related side effects include
  - Anemia (especially in African-American males)
  - Altered liver function tests/hepatotoxicity
  - Liver damage with death (very rare—may occur with flutamide)
  - Decreased libido, gynecomastia, breast tenderness, erectile dysfunction, loss of body hair and hot flashes
- Length of neoadjuvant hormonal therapy unclear.

PSYCHOSOCIAL ISSUES

- Issues including fear of radiation treatments, side effects, altered sexuality, cancer diagnosis, and its impact on family and job may all be concerns.
- Assess impact of cancer on patient and family and level of support.
- Provide support and referrals; recommend patient educational materials and resources and local support groups. Encouragement related to tolerability of therapy.
- Provide education including treatment planning process, issue of radioactivity and fear of exposing others to radiation, radiation schedule, side effect management, and tolerability of treatment.

PSA OUTCOMES AND MONITORING[29, 30]

- PSA levels should fall to < 1.0 ng/dL after treatment, but this may take several years to occur.
- First PSA should be done < 6 weeks after treatment completed and then every 3 months for 2 years, then every 6 months for 3 more years.
- ASTRO definition of PSA failure is three consecutive PSA elevations above nadir that continue to rise indicate biochemical failure and disease activity.[29]
- The failure date is the midpoint between the nadir and the first of the three consecutive PSA elevations according to the ASTRO definition.[29]
- "PSA bounce" is common after radiation therapy and occurs in 10–20% of patients after external beam radiation therapy. It is benign in etiology and does not reflect active disease. It usually falls to a level at or below the previous PSA value in 3–6 months.[29]
- A PSA bounce is most likely to occur in the first 2 years after radiation therapy is completed.

I thank Heidi Volpe, MSN, RN, CCRA, for her review of this chapter.

References

1. Hilderley LJ. Radiotherapy. In: Groenwald SL, Frogge MH, Goodman M, Yarbro CH, eds. *Cancer Nursing Principles and Practice*. 4th ed. Sudbury, Mass: Jones and Bartlett; 1997:247–282.

2. Marks S. *Prostate and Cancer: A Family Guide to Diagnosis, Treatment and Survival*. Tucson, Ariz: Fisher Books; 1997.

3. Catalona WJ. Management of cancer of the prostate [review]. *N Engl J Med*. 1994; 331:996–1004.

4. Asbell SO, Krall JM, Pilepich MV, et al. Elective pelvic irradiation in stages A2, B carcinoma of the prostate: Analysis of RTOG 77–06. *Int J Radiat Oncol Biol Phys*.1988;15:1307–1316.

5. Hanks GE, Asbell SO, Krall JM, et al. Outcome for lymph node dissection negative T1b, T2 (A-2, B) prostate cancer treated with external beam radiation therapy in RTOG 77–06. *Int J Radiat Oncol Biol Phys*. 1991;21:1099–1103.

6. Oesterling J, Fuks Z, Lee CT, Scher HI. Cancer of the prostate. In: DeVita VT, Hellman S, Rosenberg SA, eds. *Cancer: Principles and Practice of Oncology*. 5th ed. Philadelphia, Pa: Lippincott-Raven; 1997:1322–1386.

7. Scher HI, Leibel SA, Fuks Z, et al. Cancer of the prostate. In: DeVita VT, Hellman S, Rosenberg SA, eds. *Cancer: Principles and Practice of Oncology*. 7th ed. Philadelphia, Pa: Lippincott Williams & Wilkins; 2005:1192–1259.

8. Zelefsky MJ, Valicenti RK, Goodman K, Perez, CA. Prostate cancer. In: Perez CA, Brady LW, Halperin EC, Ullrich RK, eds. *Principles and Practice of Radiation Oncology*. 4th ed. Philadelphia, Pa: Lippincott Williams & Wilkins; 2004:1692–1762.

9. DeAngelis LM. Neuromuscular complications. In: Casciato DA, ed. *Manual of Clinical Oncology*. 5th ed. Philadelphia, Pa: Lippincott Williams & Wilkins; 2004:607–621.

10. Valicenti RK, Gomella LG, Ismail M, et al. The efficacy of early adjuvant therapy for pT3N0 prostate cancer: a matched pair analysis. *Int J Radiation Oncol Biol Phys*. 1999;45:53–58.

11. Anscher MS, Robertson CN, Prosnitz LR. Adjuvant radiotherapy for pathologic stage T3/4 adenocarcinoma of the prostate: Ten-year update. *Int J Radiat Oncol Biol Phys*. 1995;33:37–43.

12. Bucci MK, Bevan A, Roach M. Advances in radiation therapy: conventional to 3D, to IMRT, to 4D and beyond. *CA Cancer J Clin*. 2005;55:117–134.

13. Michalski JM, Purdy JA, Winter K, et al. Preliminary report of toxicity following 3D radiation therapy for prostate cancer on 3DOG/RTOG 94–06. *Int J Radiat Oncol Biol Phys*. 2000;46:391–402.

14. Maher KE. Male genitourinary cancers. In: Dow KH, Bucholtz JD, Iwamoto R, et al, eds. *Nursing Care in Radiation Oncology*. 2nd ed. Philadelphia, Pa: WB Saunders; 1997:184–219.

15. Perez CA. Prostate. In: Perez CA, Brady LW, eds. *Principles and Practice of Radiation Oncology*. 3rd ed. Philadelphia, Pa: Lippincott-Raven; 1998:1583–1694.

16. *Nursing 2005 Drug Handbook*. Philadelphia, Pa: Lippincott Williams & Wilkins; 2005.

17. Wilkes GM, Barton-Burke M. *2005 Oncology Nursing Drug Handbook*. Sudbury, Mass: Jones and Bartlett Publishers; 2005.

18. Sitton E. Managing side effects of skin changes and fatigue. In: Dow KH, Bucholtz JD., Iwamoto R, et al, eds. *Nursing Care in Radiation Oncology*. 2nd ed. Philadelphia, Pa: WB Saunders; 1997:79–100.

19. Marks LB, Carroll PR, Dugan TC, Anscher MS. The response of the urinary bladder, urethra, and ureter to radiation and chemotherapy. *Int J Radiat Oncol Biol Phys*. 1995;31:1257–1280.

20. Abel LJ, Blatt HJ, Stipetich RL, et al. Nursing management of patients receiving brachytherapy for early stage prostate cancer. *Clin J Oncol Nurs.* 1999;3:7–15.
21. Wernicke GA, Valicenti R, DiEva K, et al. Radiation dose delivered to the proximal penis as a predictor of the risk of erectile dysfunction after three-dimensional conformal radiotherapy for localized prostate cancer. *Int J Radiat Oncol Biol Phys.* 2004;60:1357–1363.
22. DuPen AR, Panke JT. Common clinical problems. In: Varricchio C, Pierce M, Walker CL, Ades TB, eds. *A Cancer Source Book for Nurses.* 7th ed. Sudbury, Mass: Jones and Bartlett; 1997:174–184.
23. Asbell SO, Leon SA, Tester WJ, et al. Development of anemia and recovery in prostate cancer patients treated with combined androgen blockade and radiotherapy. *Prostate.* 1996;29:243–248.
24. Lynch MP, Jacobs LA. The assessment and diagnosis of anemia in the patient with cancer. Newtown, PA: Associates in Medical Marketing, 1998. Anemia and Fatigue in Cancer Patients: Nursing Care Management. Philadelphia, Pa: Nursing symposium, April 1997.
25. Garnick MB. Hormonal therapy in the management of prostate cancer: From Huggins to the present. *Urology.* 1997;49(suppl 3A):5–15.
26. Roach M. Neoadjuvant total androgen suppression and radiotherapy in the management of locally advanced prostate cancer. *Semin Urol Oncol.* 1996;14:32–38.
27. Pilepich MV, Caplan R, Byhardt RW, et al. Phase III trial of adjuvant androgen suppression using goserelin in patients with carcinoma of the prostate treated with definitive radiotherapy: Results of 85–31 [abstract]. *Int J Radiat Oncol Biol Phys.* 1995;32:188.
28. Zelefsky MJ, Harrison A. Neoadjuvant androgen ablation prior to radiotherapy for prostate cancer: reducing the potential morbidity of therapy. *Urology.* 1997;49:38–45.
29. American Society for Therapeutic Radiology and Oncology Consensus Panel. Consensus statement: Guidelines for PSA following radiation therapy. *Int J Radiat Oncol Biol Phys.* 1997;37:1035.
30. Rossner CJ, Kuban DA, Levy LA, et al. The prostate-specific antigen bounce phenomenon after external beam radiation for clinically localized prostate cancer. *J Urol.* 2002;168:2001–2005.

Interstitial Brachytherapy

EVOLUTION OF PROSTATIC BRACHYTHERAPY[1-6]
- Radioactive material is placed in the prostate tissue to treat prostate cancer.
- With the advent of CT scanners and TRUS, computer-based treatment planning became possible and common.
- Materials used for brachytherapy include iodine-125 (I-125) and palladium-103 (Pd-103) in the form of implants.
- Additional advances and improvements included implant technique (peripheral seed loading), use of ultrasound guidance, and treatment planning computers.
- Result has been better patient outcomes in terms of optimal radiation dosing and less bowel, bladder, and erectile toxicity.

ELIGIBILITY CRITERIA/EXCLUSION CRITERIA
- As a single form of therapy—organ-confined disease as evidenced by clinical stage of ≤ T2a, Gleason score ≤ 6, PSA < 10, and low volume of disease[2, 5, 7, 8]
- Possible exclusion criteria—age > 80; pubic arch interference; > 50 cc prostate volume; median lobe hypertrophy; high American Urologic Association urinary score; chronic urinary obstructive symptoms; history of TURP[5, 6]
- Additional therapies may be added such as external beam radiation therapy (EBRT) or hormonal therapy. Hormonal therapy may be used before, during, or after brachytherapy and/or concurrently with brachytherapy. EBRT can be used before or after brachytherapy with or without hormonal therapy.
- The following variables are considered important in the decision-making process for recommending brachytherapy alone or in combination with EBRT with or without hormonal therapy: large prostate volume producing urinary symptoms, Gleason score ≥ 7, PSA > 10, adverse clinical or pathologic criteria[5, 6, 9-11]

BIOCHEMICAL OUTCOMES
- PSA is used to monitor patients for residual or relapsed disease.
- Goal is PSA ≤ 0.5 ng/mL (nadir). May take as long as 5 years (or longer) to be attained.[2, 5, 8-10]
- Patient is monitored every 4–6 months for 5 years and then usually yearly thereafter.[12]
- American Society of Therapeutic Radiology and Oncology (ASTRO) consensus panel recommendation for failure determination: After the nadir has been reached, three consecutive increases in the PSA are required. The date of failure is the midpoint between the nadir and the first date of the PSA increase.[12] These guidelines are under revision due to the ambiguity of PSA readings after treatment.
- Other methods of patient monitoring include PSA doubling time and PSA velocity.
- Temporary PSA rise or bump often occurs 12–36 months postimplant in 30–50% of patients.[5, 13]

- Options for patients who are brachytherapy "failures" include EBRT; use of a different implantable isotope or retreating with brachytherapy; surgery, hormonal therapy, or cryosurgery[5, 6, 14]
- Over 90% of patients with low-risk disease have biochemical freedom from disease progression for 10 years. For patients with intermediate- and high-grade disease, who are treated with brachytherapy and EBRT *with or without* hormonal therapy, 65–79% are disease free.[2–5, 9]

TYPES OF PERMANENT SEEDS

- Pd-103 and I-125 are commonly used low-energy photon emitters with different half-lives and different side effect profiles due to the half-life and photon energy differences.[6]
- Pd-103 half-life is 17 days.[6]
- I-125 half-life is 60 days, available mounted on suture material, which may allow for easier placement, reduced risk of seed migration, and greater flexibility during placement procedure.[5, 15]

THE PROCEDURE

- Bowel preparation begins day before and continues in morning preprocedure. May include enemas, laxatives, clear liquids or full-liquid diet for 24 hours preprocedure and NPO status.
- Blood work and tests: CBC, PT/INR/PTT, chemistry panel, urine analysis, chest X-ray, EKG, CT scan, ultrasound (volume study) or MRI
- May be done as an outpatient procedure
- Anesthesia—local, general, or spinal
- Pre-op meds—antibiotics, anti-inflammatories, alpha-blockers
- Treatment planning—Each patient has a seed implant treatment plan.
- Procedure—anchoring to prevent gland from moving,[6, 7] needles with implant inserted through a perineal template or by using transperineal ultrasound[5, 6, 14, 16]
- Cystourethroscopy is performed to retrieve misplaced seeds or blood clots after seed placement procedure is completed.
- Indwelling urinary drainage catheter—monitor urinary output, allows for bladder irrigation
- Side effect prevention—careful positioning, DVT prophylaxis, antibiotics, corticosteroids
- Most patients are discharged the same day or hospitalized overnight for observation. The indwelling urinary catheter is usually removed before discharge.
- Precaution—seeds may migrate to retroperitoneum, veins, bladder, urethra, heart, lungs. Rarely does this affect treatment to the prostate.[5, 6, 14, 17, 18]

SIDE EFFECTS

Urinary

- Mild to moderate intensity, expected, acute
- Frequency, urgency, hesitancy, hematuria, dysuria, nocturia, decreased flow of stream[5, 19–22]
- Duration dependent on isotope source used (longer for iodine than for palladium)
- Hematuria is caused by needles and seed placement; lasts 24–72 hours. May continue or recur due to prostatitis.[5, 20–22] Hematuria lasting longer than 6 months may have a different etiology and requires a urologic evaluation.

- Urinary retention is due to clots, inflammation of prostate from seeds causing it to increase in size, postoperative edema. Occurs 24–28 hours postprocedure[5, 19, 20, 22]

Managed with preventative medications—antibiotics (parenteral and oral) for 3–7 days; nonsteroidal anti-inflammatories (NSAIDs)—for days to weeks; anxiolytics/sedatives—for days to weeks; alpha-blockers—for several weeks to months. If, in spite of this regimen, urinary retention develops, urinary catheterization is performed (indwelling or intermittent self-catheterization).

- In patients with prior TURP, higher incidence of urinary incontinence
- Patients should not smoke or use tobacco as their usage delays wound healing and interferes with restoration of urinary tract function.[21]

Bowel

- Proctitis, constipation, diarrhea, rectal bleeding is usually minimal, may be related to hemorrhoids, manipulation of rectum during implant procedure, or medications.
- Proctitis may last weeks to months.
- Rectal bleeding—Radiation may make rectal tissue more fragile[5, 22–24]; rectal bleeding may persist or recur 6–18 months after implant procedure. Medications that may be effective include oral sucralfate, steroid or mesalamine suppositories, or enemas. A gastroenterology evaluation may be needed for coagulation therapies.[5, 25, 26] If rectal wall biopsy is performed, the patient may develop rectal ulcers or fistulas.[5, 23, 27]

Erectile Dysfunction

- Common and permanent to some degree
- Potency rates at 6 years—39–70%[5, 9, 14, 28]
- Multiple other variables affect potency, not just the cancer therapy.
- Medications[5, 14, 28–31]
- PDE5 inhibitors—92% effective. Common side effects are headache, nasal stuffiness, flushing, GI upset, and vision changes. Drug interactions—nitrates, alpha-blockers, illegal drugs.
- Intraurethral alprostadil
- Intracavernosal injections
- Penile implants
- Cause of erectile dysfunction could be related to damage to the vasculature or nerves, but more research is needed.[5, 14, 32–34] It is hoped recent advances in localization and effective radiation blocking techniques for penile bulb and vessels and tissues will reduce incidence.
- Other side effects are bloody ejaculate; discolored, reduced or dry ejaculate; or temporary oligospermia.[5, 14, 29, 32, 33]

SYMPTOM MANAGEMENT/PATIENT EDUCATION (see Table 11–1 and Table 11–2)

Patient Education

- Procedures: preimplant—anesthesia, tests; implant; postimplant
- Symptom management
- Radiation safety
  - Institution/facility/regulatory agency-dependent related to straining urine for seeds, seed retrieval, or flushing. Keeping required distances from other people. For adults: Pd-103—minimal restrictions on adult contact. I-125—must keep several feet from adults for several months. There are lead-lined aprons and undergarments available that when worn loosen this restriction.[5]

- For contact with children and pregnant women: I-125 patients *must* avoid prolonged and close proximity contact for 1–2 months unless wearing lead-lined undergarments or lap shields. Pd-103 patients *must* avoid prolonged and close proximity for 3–4 weeks.
- Medication regimen and prescriptions and instructions, follow-up, when to call physician
- Use of ice packs and sitz baths for pain management
- Patient should expect moderate bruising, mild perineal tenderness, urinary/ voiding changes, need to take medications as prescribed (antibiotics, alpha-blockers, steroids/NSAIDs) to prevent infection, improve urinary flow by relaxing smooth muscles, and decreasing inflammation. Some rectal discomfort (use mesalamine or steroid suppositories) occurs. Bloody, discolored, and reduced ejaculate[5, 22]
- Diet—low fiber, drink plenty of fluids
- Avoid bladder irritants—alcohol, caffeine, citrus, over-the-counter vitamins, and supplements[5, 22]
- Activity—avoid activity that places pressure on perineal area (riding a horse, bicycle, motorcycle, tractor, lawn mower, etc.). Avoid hot tubs > 100^0F.[5, 22]
- Sexual activity—condom required for 1 month for Pd-103 and 2 or more months for I-125.[5, 22]

NURSING ASSESSMENT OF BOWEL, URINARY, AND SEXUAL FUNCTIONING

Intraoperative nursing management—safety, radiation safety, medications, supportive care, catheter care

Postoperative care—anesthesia precautions, urinary function, care of indwelling urinary catheter, bladder irrigation, medication administration, pain management

Assessment of emotional impact of disease and treatment on patient, spouse, and family

TEMPORARY HIGH–DOSE RATE (HDR) IMPLANTS

- Often used with EBRT, before, during, or after HDR. Benefits of combined radiation therapy may include: shorter EBRT treatment schedule, less radiation exposure to staff, better radiation delivery[6, 34, 35]
- Candidates include patients with T1b to T3b disease, no distant metastases, no large TURP defects, gland volume < 80 cm.[3, 5, 6]
- Catheters are placed in the prostate through the perineum using ultrasound to guide catheter placement. CT scan done to plan treatment, and patient has radiation delivered intermittently via the catheters over a period of 24–36 hours. Two treatments are often given daily each separated by 6 hours. Treatment is done in the radiation therapy department or under anesthesia in the OR. Iridium-192 is placed in the catheters by a device designed to administer this type of therapy. The treatment takes about 25 minutes each time. Between treatments, the patient is not radioactive as the source is removed at the end of each treatment. The patient is returned to his hospital bed and usually discharged after 1 day.
- Outcomes/response rates[6, 35–38]
  - T1–T2—93% for HDR alone
  - T3—69–87% for HDR and EBRT administered together
- Side effects[37, 38]
  - Similar to those associated with permanent implants
  - Greater risk of incontinence, urethral stricture

TABLE 11-1 Palladium 103 Interstitial Brachytherapy Prostate Symptom Management Protocol

Side Effect		Symptoms	Interventions (for duration of symptoms)
Skin		• Bruising of scrotum/perineum • Tenderness/ discomfort • Hematoma	• Apply ice packs to perineum as needed first 24 hours as a comfort measure and to reduce local swelling • Sitz baths 2–3 times daily as a comfort measure • Avoid hot tub temp (< 100°F recommeded) as a comfort measure • Mild analgesics (ibuprofen, acetaminophen) as a comfort measure

Urinary	Acute	• Frequency
		• Urgency
		• Hesitancy
		• Hematuria
		• Dysuria
		• Bladder spasms (uncommon)
		• Incomplete bladder emptying
		• Nocturia
			• Alpha-blockers (titrate dose)
			  Tamsulosin 0.4 mg 1–2 x day
			  Doxazosin 1–8 mg qd
			  Terazosin 1–10 mg qd
			  Alfuzosin 10 mg qd
			Educate patient about potential hypotensive episodes, dizziness, GI upset peripheral edema[40]
			• Steroids vs. NSAIDs—educate about peripheral edema, blood pressure changes, blood sugar changes[40]
			• Avoid dietary bladder irritants (coffee, tea, alcohol, citrus) as a comfort measure
			• Increase water intake to maintain urine dilution and reduce dysuria
			• Limit fluids after 8 p.m. to reduce nocturia
			• Antispasmodics (for bladder spasms)
			  Tolterodine tartate 2–4 mg qd
			  Oxybutynin chloride 5–15 mg qd
			  Belladonna and opium suppository q12 hours
			  Educate about dry mouth, constipation, somnolence, risk of urinary retention/infection[40]
			• Urinary antiseptics (combination products that include methylene blue)—educate patient about discoloration of urine, rash, flushing of skin, dizziness.[40]
			• Urinary alkalinzers—potassium citrate, sodium bicarbonate. Educate about GI upset, bowel changes, electrolyte disturbance.[40]

continues

TABLE 11-1 Palladium 103 Interstitial Brachytherapy Prostate Symptom Management Protocol, continued

Side Effect		Symptoms	Interventions (for duration of symptoms)
Urinary, cont'd		• Urinary retention	• Activity modification. Avoid bicycle or motorcycle riding, long periods of sitting
			• Perform voiding trial
			• Phenoxybenzamine hydrochloride or bethanecol chloride tid (typically several weeks) to increase urine flow. Educate about hypotensive episodes, bowel changes, flushing of skin.
			• Indwelling catheter vs. teaching intermittent self-catheterization
	Late	• Dysuria • Hematuria	• Avoid dietary bladder irritants.
			• Urinary alkalinizers
			• Increase water intake.
			• Pentosan polysulfate sodium 100 mg tid for 6–12 months to reduce symptoms of chronic dysuria. Educate about GI upset, bowel changes.
			• Antidepressants/anxiolytic—amitriptyline hydrochloride 25–50 mg qhs or alprazolam 0.25–0.5 mg qhs. Educate about drowsiness, dizziness, and caution with driving and operating heavy equipment.[40]
			* Dimethyl sulfoxide (DMSO) bladder installations for chronic dysuria/cystitis, not remedied by other medications. Educate about garlic odor on breath and skin, and possible transient discomfort during installation.[40]
			• Other workup: urine cytology, IVP, cystoscopy, Nuclear Matrix Protein (NMP-22) to determine etiology of chronic hematuria
			• If workup negative for bladder or kidney disease, institute finasteride 5 mg qd x 6–12 months. Educate about decreased potency, libido, decreased volume of ejaculate, and depression of PSA level.[40]
Rectal	Acute	• Bowel changes • Looseness/ constipation	• Low-residue diet
			• Sitz baths as needed

Rectal, cont'd	Acute	• Frequency • Urgency • Painless rectal bleeding • Rectal irritation	• Sucralfate 1 gm 4–6x day to regulate bowel consistency; protect rectal mucosa. Educate about GI upset • Hydrocortisone or mesalamine suppository 1–2x day to reduce rectal discomfort. To be used 6 weeks or less. Educate about bowel changes.[40] • Nonprescriptive fiber laxatives to reduce incidence of diarrhea or constipation • Avoidance of rectal manipulation for 8–12 months to reduce aggravating effects to existing rectal symptoms
	Late	• Proctitis • Bleeding • Rectal discomfort	• Mesalamine suppository qd • Sucralfate 1 gm 4–6x days • Pentoxifylline 400 mg tid to reduce incidence of rectal bleeding and aid in healing of tissue. Educate about GI upset, dizziness, headache. [40] • Colonoscopy to evaluate chronic rectal bleeding not remedied by medications • Laser coagulation to remedy chronic rectal bleeding not resolved by medications

Erectile dysfunction	Acute & Late	• Decreased ability to maintain erection	• Address psychogenic causes (e.g., stress, marital problems, job responsibilities, etc.)
			• PDE5 inhibitors (sildenafil, vardenafil, tadalafil)—educate about contraindication of nitrates, visual changes, headache, nasal stuffiness, possible interaction with alpha-blockers, prolonged erection[40]
			• Alprostadil intraurethral suppositories—educate about penile irritation, urethritis[40]
			• Intracavernosal alprostadil self-injections—educate about penile pain, prolonged erection, hematoma[40]
			  • Vacuum erection device (requires prescription)
			   • OTC supplements (no testosterone derivative)
			Supplements do not increase testosterone levels, but enhance body's ability to utilize existing testosterone levels

Source: Courtesy of Dattoli Cancer Center and Research Institute, Sarasota, Florida. Used with permission.

TABLE 11-2 Standard of Nursing Practice for Prostate Brachytherapy

Nursing Diagnosis	Outcome	Nursing Interventions
Knowledge deficit related to prostate brachytherapy procedure	The patient will be able to verbalize understanding of the prostate brachytherapy procedure and self-care measures postprocedure. The patient will promptly notify the health care provider of any significant postoperative symptoms.	• Assess patient's baseline understanding of the brachytherapy procedure. • Identify and address misconceptions, and provide education as to preoperative procedures, intraoperative procedures, and postoperative care. • Provide education as to self-care measures, expected postprocedure side effects, complications, and significant problems/issues/symptoms to report to health care provider.
Potential for altered urinary elimination secondary to postoperative prostate inflammation or bleeding with clot formation interfering with voiding	The patient will be able to verbalize understanding of expected postoperative inflammation to prostate causing expected urinary symptoms, the need for adherence to prescribed medications, and an understanding of when to notify health care provider if unable to urinate within a specified time frame postprocedure.	• Review patient's preexisting urinary function and related medical conditions prior to procedure. • Educate patient of importance of adhering to prescribed medications postprocedure despite level of urinary symptoms. • Educate patient to ensure adequate fluid intake, and to measure intake and output as necessary if discomfort ensues. • Educate patient as to importance of avoidance of dietary bladder irritants that may aggravate urinary function. • Assess patient's understanding of need to notify health care provider and/or seek emergent medical attention if inability to urinate lasts greater than a specified period of time. • If patient sent home with indwelling urinary catheter or taught intermittent self-catheterization, assess patient's understanding of how to take care of catheter and when to perform self-catheterization.

TABLE 11–2 Standard of Nursing Practice for Prostate Brachytherapy, continued

Nursing Diagnosis	Outcome	Nursing Interventions
Potential for alteration in bowel elimination related to anesthesia, post-operative medications, and procedural rectal manipulation	The patient will verbalize understanding of expected postoperative bowel changes and identify significant changes in bowel function requiring the need to contact health care provider.	• Review patient's preexisting bowel function and related medical conditions prior to procedure. • Educate patient of importance of adhering to prescribed medications despite level of change of bowel function. • Educate patient as to when to notify health care provider for prolonged constipation, diarrhea, increased rectal bleeding. • Educate patient as to importance of adequate fluid intake. • Educate patient as to importance of diet, low residue versus high residue, dependent upon symptoms. • Educate patient as to avoidance of any rectal manipulation per physician order for a specified time frame.
Risk for sexual dysfunction related to disease or post-treatment sequelae	Patient will verbalize understanding of temporary and potentially permanent erectile dysfunction and/or libido postbrachytherapy.	• Address psychogenic causes (i.e., stress, marital problems, job responsibilities, etc.) and refer as necessary for counseling. • Assess associated physiologic causes of impotence pretreatment (diabetes, hypertension, alcohol, tobacco, aging, etc.) and educate patient on behavior modification where possible (cessation of smoking, reduce alcohol consumption). • Educate patient as to radiation-related erectile dysfunction and expected time frame of dysfunction. • Educate patient (and significant other) as to medical interventions available to be used during period of dysfunction.

Source: Cash JC. Interstitial brachytherapy. In: Held-Warmkessel, J., ed. *Contemporary Issues in Prostate Cancer: A Nursing Perspective* (2nd ed). Jones and Bartlett Publishers, 2006, 229–247. Reprinted with permission by Jones and Bartlett Publishers.

- Nursing care issues/symptom management [39]
  - Pre-op—bowel prep, pretesting, ultrasound, patient education (epidural anesthesia, procedure, hospitalization)
  - Intraoperative care—monitoring patient for urethral bleeding and bladder spasms, providing catheter care, patient positioning for comfort and to reduce musculoskeletal discomfort
  - Post-op care
    - Clear liquid to low residue diet
    - Pain management
    - Antiemetics, antidiarrheals, antibiotics
    - Continuous bladder irrigation
    - Indwelling urinary catheter care (removed 24 hours after perineal catheters)
    - Maintaining sterile dressing to perineal area after catheters removed
    - Sitz baths and analgesics for pain management
    - Side effects—perineal pain responds to steroids or NSAIDs; urinary and rectal symptoms last several weeks to months

I thank Jennifer Cash, MS, ARNP, OCN®, for her review of this chapter.

References

1. Holm HH, Juul N, Pederse JF, et al. Transperineal iodine-125 seed implantation in prostate cancer guided by transrectal ultrasonography. *Journal of Urology.* 1983; 130:283–286.

2. Ragde H, Blasko J, Grimm P, et al. Interstitial iodine-125 radiation without adjuvant therapy in the treatment of clinically localized prostate carcinoma. *Cancer.* 1997; 80:442–453.

3. Abel L, Dafoe-Lambie J, Butler W, et al. Treatment outcomes and quality of life issues for patients treated with prostate brachytherapy. *Clin J Oncol Nurs.* 2003; 7:48–54.

4. Ragde H, Grado GL, Nadir BS. Brachytherapy for clinically localized prostate cancer: thirteen year disease-free survival of 769 consecutive prostate cancer patients treated with permanent implants alone. *Arch Esp Urol.* 2001;54:739–747.

5. Wallner K, Blasko J, Dattoli M. *Brachytherapy Made Complicated.* 2nd ed. Washington, DC: SmartMedicine Press; 2001;5–377.

6. Perez CA, Brady LW, Halperin EC, et al. *Principles and Practice of Radiation Oncology.* 4th ed. Philadelphia, Pa: Lippincott, Williams & Wilkins; 2004:604–635, 1692–1762.

7. Zelefsky MJ, Wallner KE, Ling CC, et al. Comparison of the 5 year outcomes and morbidity of three-dimensional radiotherapy versus transperineal permanent iodine-125 implant for early stage prostate cancer. *J Clin Oncol.* 1999; 17:517–522.

8. Merrick GS, Butler WM, Galbreath RW, et al. Five year biochemical outcome following permanent interstitial brachytherapy for clinical T1-T3 prostate cancer. *Int J Radiat Oncol Biol Phys.* 2001;51:41–48.

9. Dattoli M, Wallner K, True L, et al. Long-term outcomes after treatment with external beam radiation and palladium-103 for patients with higher risk prostate carcinoma. *Cancer.* 2003;97:1–5.

10. Merrick GS, Butler WM, Lief JH, et al. Biochemical outcome for hormone-naive intermediate risk prostate cancer managed with permanent interstitial brachytherapy and supplemental external beam radiation. *Brachytherapy.* 2002;1:95–101.

11. Blasko JC, Grimm PD, Sylvester JE, et al. The role of external beam radiotherapy with I-125/Pd-103 brachytherapy for prostate carcinoma. *Radiotherapeutic Oncol.* 2000;57:273–278.

12. American Society for Therapeutic Radiology and Oncology. Guidelines for PSA following radiation therapy. *Int J Radiat Oncol Biol Phys.* 1997;37:1035–1041.

13. Cavanagh W, Blasko JC, Grimm PD, et al. Transient elevation of serum prostate-specific antigen following I-125/Pd-103 brachytherapy for localized prostate cancer. *Sem Urol Oncol.* 2000;18:160–165.

14. Dattoli MJ. *Palladium Brachytherapy: Rationale, Design and Evaluation.* Sarasota, Fla: Dattoli Cancer Foundation; 2004:5–46.

15. Butler WM, Merrick GS. I-125 RAPID Strand loading technique. *Radiat Oncol Invest.* 1996;4:48–49.

16. Peschel RE, Chen Z, Roberts K, et al. Long-term complications with prostate implants: iodine-125 vs. palladium-103. *Radiat Oncol Invest.* 1999;7:278–288.

17. Nag S, Vivekanandam S, Martinez-Monge, R. Pulmonary embolization of permanently implanted radioactive palladium-103 seeds for carcinoma of the prostate. *Int J Radiat Oncol Biol Phys.* 1997;39:667–670.

18. Tapen EM, Blasko JC, Grimm, PD. Reduction of radioactive seed embolization to the lung following prostate brachytherapy. *Int J Radiat Oncol Biol Phys.* 1998;42:1063–1067.

19. Merrick GS, Butler WM, Lief JH, et al. Temporal resolution of urinary morbidity following prostate brachytherapy. *Int J Radiat Oncol Biol Phys.* 2000;47:121–128.

20. Stone NN, Stock RG. Complications following permanent prostate brachytherapy. *Eur Urol.* 2002;41:427–433.

21. Merrick GS, Butler WM, Wallner KE, et al. Long-term urinary quality of life after permanent prostate brachytherapy. *Int J Radiat Oncol Biol Phys.* 2003;56:454–461.

22. Cash JC, Dattoli, MJ. Management of patients receiving transperineal palladium-103 prostate implants. *Oncol Nurs Forum.* 1997;24:1361–1367.

23. Merrick GS, Butler WM, Dorsey AT, et al. Rectal function following prostate brachytherapy. *Int J Radiat Oncol Biol Phys.* 1998;41:263–265.

24. Hu K, Wallner, K. Clinical course of rectal bleeding following I-125 prostate brachytherapy. *Int J Radiat Oncol Biol Phys.* 1998;41:263–265.

25. Viggiano TR, Zighelboim J, Ahlquist DA, et al. Endoscopic Nd: YAG laser coagulation of bleeding from radiation proctopathy. *Gastrointest Endosc.* 2000;39:513–517.

26. Roche B, Chautems R, Marti, MC. Application of formaldehyde for treatment of hemorrhagic radiation-induced proctitis. *World J Surg.* 1996;20:1092–1095.

27. Theodorescu D, Gillenwater JY, Koutrouvelis PG. Prostatourethral-rectal fistula after prostate brachytherapy. *Cancer.* 2000;89:2085–2091.

28. Merrick GS, Butler WM, Galbreath RW, et al. Erectile function after permanent prostatic brachytherapy. *Int J Radiat Oncol Biol Phys.* 2002;52:893–902.

29. Merrick GS, Wallner K, Butler WM, et al. Short term sexual function after prostate brachytherapy. *Int J Cancer.* 2001;96:313–319.

30. Zelefsky MJ, McKee AB, Lee H, et al. Efficacy of oral sildenafil in patients with erectile dysfunction after radiotherapy for carcinoma of the prostate. *Urology.* 1999;53:775–778.

31. Merrick GS, Wallner K, Butler WM. Management of sexual dysfunction after prostate brachytherapy. *Oncology (Huntington).* 2003;17:52–62.

32. Zelefsky MJ, Eid, JF. Elucidating the etiology of erectile dysfunction after definitive therapy for prostatic cancer. *Int J Radiat Oncol Biol Phys.* 1998;40:129–133.

33. Merrick GS, Butler WM, Dorsey AT, et al. A comparison of radiation dose to the neurovascular bundles in men with and without prostate brachytherapy induced erectile dysfunction. *Int J Radiat Oncol Biol Phys*. 2000;48:1069–1074.

34. Merrick GS, Butler WM, Wallner K, et al. The importance of radiation doses to the penile bulb vs. crura in the development of postbrachytherapy erectile dysfunction. *Int J Radiat Oncol Biol Phys*. 2002;54:1055–1062.

35. Vicini F, Vargas C, Gustafson G, et al. High dose rate brachytherapy in the treatment of prostate cancer. *World J Urol*. 2003;21:220–228.

36. Grills JS, Martinez AA, Hollander M, . High dose rate brachytherapy as prostate cancer monotherapy reduces toxicity compared to low dose palladium seeds. *J Urol*. 2004;171:1098–1104.

37. Deger S, Boehmer D, Turk I, et al. High dose rate brachytherapy for local prostate cancer. *Eur Urol*. 2002;41:420–426.

38. Syed AM, Puthawala A, Sharma A, et al. High dose rate brachytherapy in the treatment of carcinoma of the prostate. *Cancer Contr*. 2001;8:511–521.

39. Colella J, Scrofine S. High dose rate brachytherapy for treating prostate cancer: nursing considerations. *Urol Nurs*. 2004;24:39–44.

40. Physician's Desk Reference. *Urology Prescribing Guide*. 5th ed. Tokyo, Japan: Yamanouchi Pharmaceutical Co., Ltd; 2004:5–35,243–345.

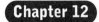

Hormonal Therapy

INTRODUCTION

Uses[1]

- Management of metastatic prostate cancer
- Neoadjuvant or adjuvant therapy with radiation therapy or surgery

RATIONALE FOR HORMONAL MANIPULATION[1-14]

- Hypothalamic-pituitary-testicular axis regulates prostate cell growth.
- Hormones are released from these organs in pulses.
- Luteinizing hormone-releasing hormone (LHRH) is manufactured by the arcuate nucleus of the hypothalamus.
- LHRH causes pituitary gonadotrophin receptors to make and release luteinizing hormone (LH) and follicle stimulating hormone (FSH).
- Controlled by hormonal feedback
- LH results in testosterone production.
- Testosterone is converted to dihydrotestosterone (DHT) in prostate by enzyme 5α-reductase.
- DHT controls prostate cell growth and function.
- DHT binds to androgen receptor (AR) and binds to DNA.
- Binding causes gene expression controlling androgen-receptive growth.
- Adrenal glands produce weak sex steroids that are converted to DHT in the prostate, with approximately 10–40% of the resulting intraprostatic DHT being of adrenal origin.
- Hormonal manipulation goal—stop androgen-dependent prostate cell growth and induce apoptosis.
- With loss of androgens, prostate cell death begins in 24 hours.

PRIMARY HORMONAL MANIPULATION[1, 14, 15, 22-25]

Introduction

- First method of treating metastatic prostate cancer
- Accomplished surgically or medically
- Side effects of androgen deprivation include
  - Loss of libido
  - Impotence
  - Fatigue
  - Hot flashes
  - Weight redistribution
  - Muscle atrophy
  - Osteoporosis
  - Cognitive dysfunction
  - Decreased HDL
- See **Table 12–1** for hormone therapy standard of care.[15-21]

TABLE 12–1 Hormonal Therapy Standard of Care

NURSING DIAGNOSIS: Testosterone suppression related to hormonal therapy

OUTCOME: Serum testosterone level falls to castrate level (< 50 mg/dL). PSA level will be decreased • Pt will verbalize reduction in symptoms

NURSING INTERVENTION: Monitor serum testosterone levels • Educate patient as to need to adhere to plan of follow-up surveillance as recommended by physician such as PSA, physical exam with DRE, and diagnostic studies such as bone scan

NURSING DIAGNOSIS: Knowledge deficit related to hormonal therapy

OUTCOME: Pt will verbalize understanding of rationale for treatment with hormonal manipulation, goals of treatment, potential side effects, and interventions to minimize side effects

NURSING INTERVENTION: Assess patient's understanding of goals of hormonal therapy and potential side effects and their management • Educate as appropriate, providing repetition and clarification as needed • Provide additional informational support and other resources such as National Cancer Institute (1-800-4-cancer) and American Cancer Society, prostate cancer support groups

NURSING DIAGNOSIS: Altered body image related to side effects of therapy such as hot flashes, fatigue, altered sexual functioning

OUTCOME: Pt will verbalize an acceptable level of self-esteem and self-image

NURSING INTERVENTION: Assess patient's response to effects of treatment that affect body image
• Encourage verbalization of feelings • Encourage pt to participate in support groups, if appropriate

OUTCOME: Pt will have tolerable level of discomfort related to hot flashes

NURSING INTERVENTION: Assess pt for incidence, frequency, and intensity of hot flashes
• Educate pt as to treatment options available • Assess effectiveness of intervention and need to try alternative interventions

OUTCOME: Pt will verbalize understanding of management of fatigue

NURSING INTERVENTION: Assess pt for causes of fatigue such as anemia, pain, inadequate nutrition, weight loss, inadequate rest or sleep, depression, or anxiety • Educate pt as to cause of fatigue • Encourage pt to keep a diary of fatigue and evaluate diary for patterns of fatigue • Assist pt in identifying activities that can be performed by other people
• Encourage pt to participate in preferred/favorite activities and delegate others
• Encourage program of regular exercise such as walking

OUTCOME: Pt will describe methods personally acceptable for management of erectile dysfunction

NURSING INTERVENTION: Assess pt for decreased libido and erectile dysfunction • Educate pt and significant other in treatment options for erectile dysfunction • Recognize that sexual dysfunction may be multifactorial and refer as appropriate

NURSING DIAGNOSIS: Risk for fracture related to osteoporosis

OUTCOME: Pt will not sustain a fracture

TABLE 12–1 Hormonal Therapy Standard of Care, continued

NURSING INTERVENTION: Consider supplemental calcium and vitamin D; Consider bone mineral density determination at beginning of hormonal therapy and at periodic intervals
• Consider concurrent administration of bisphosphonate to inhibit bone resorption (dependent on clinical trial outcomes) • Encourage lifestyle modifications that reduce other risk factors associated with osteoporosis; maintain normal weight for height, and no smoking. Encourage regular daily exercise and include weight-resistant exercise

NURSING DIAGNOSIS: Potential for side effects related to drug therapy such as diarrhea, interstitial lung disease, or risk for injury resulting from alcohol interaction with nilutamide

OUTCOME: Pt will verbalize understanding of diarrhea management

NURSING INTERVENTION: Educate pt as to potential drug side effects • Reduce dose of flutamide by 50% if diarrhea develops. If diarrhea does not resolve, stop flutamide and use another agent on trial basis • Educate pt to take flutamide q 8 h and not tid

OUTCOME: Pt will have prompt recognition of breathing problems

NURSING INTERVENTION: Assess pt for shortness of breath, cough, chest pain, or fever, and teach pt to notify nurse or physician immediately if they occur • Monitor pt during first 3 mo of nilutamide therapy for respiratory problems. If they develop, obtain chest radiograph, and monitor pt for interstitial changes. Stop drug if changes develop • Monitor pt to acertain that symptoms improve

OUTCOME: Pt will not drink alcohol while taking nilutamide

NURSING INTERVENTION: Educate pt as to danger of consuming alcohol while taking nilutamide

OUTCOME: Pt will not sustain injury while taking nilutamide

NURSING INTERVENTION: Educate pt to avoid night driving while taking nilutamide

---

PSA, prostate-specific antigen; PT, patient; DRE, digital rectal exam; q, every; tid, three times a day.

Data compiled from Harris et al.,[15] Portenoy and Miaskowski,[16] Stepan et al.,[17] Townsend et al.,[18] Sisson de Castro,[19] Daniell,[20] and Diamond.[21]

Source: Stempkowski L. Hormonal therapy. In: Held-Warmkessel, J., ed. *Contemporary Issues in Prostate Cancer: A Nursing Perspective* (2nd ed). Jones and Bartlett Publishers, 2006, 248–283. Reprinted with permission by Jones and Bartlett Publishers.

Medical Castration[2, 22–25]

- LHRH agonists
  - Inhibit pituitary release of LH
  - First dose results in increased level of testosterone with LH production increase—may produce disease flare with increased symptoms such as bone pain or urinary obstruction; lasts 5–8 days. Testosterone levels then fall to castration level.
  - Flare eliminated by administering an antiandrogen, such as flutamide, prior to administering LHRH agents. The exact time of starting an antiandrogen prior to LHRH agonist administration is not well defined. Antiandrogen administration should continue for 1 month after LHRH agonist administration.
  - Action of antiandrogen—block binding of testosterone to AR
  - Determine if castrate level (< 20 mg/mL) of testosterone achieved by checking blood testosterone level.

TABLE 12–2 LHRH Agonists

Drug	Formulation	Dosage
Leuprolide acetate		
Lupron	Prefilled dual-chamber syringe containing lyophilized particles for reconstitution to depot suspension for IM injection	Equivalent to 7.5 mg/mo Available in the following injections: 7.5 mg/mo 22.5 mg/3 mo 30 mg/4 mo
Eligard	Prefilled syringes for reconstitution to depot suspension for SC injection	In addition to above, a 45 mg/6 mo formulation is under FDA review
Viadur	An osmotically driven implant requiring physician placement	12-month implant
Goserelin (Zoladex)	Prepared syringe with biodegradable implant for SC injection in upper abdomen	Equivalent of 3.6 mg/mo Available in the following injections: 3.6 mg/mo 10.8 mg/mo
Histrelin (Vantas)	A flexible, hydrogel implant requiring physician placement	12-month implant

Product information, TAP Pharmaceuticals, 2003.
Product information, Sanofi~Synthelabo, 2003.
Product information, Bayer Pharmaceuticals, 2002.
Product information, Zeneca Pharmaceuticals, 2003.
Product information, Valera Pharmaceuticals, 2004.
Source: Stempkowski L. Hormonal therapy. In: Held-Warmkessel, J., ed. *Contemporary Issues in Prostate Cancer: A Nursing Perspective* (2nd ed). Jones and Bartlett Publishers, 2006, 248–283. Reprinted with permission by Jones and Bartlett Publishers.

- Adding an antiandrogen to LHRH agonist or to orchiectomy may be necessary if castrate level is not achieved.
- LHRH agents are administered by injection; frequency of administration varies by type of preparation used (see **Table 12–2**)
- LHRH antagonists
  - Block LHRH receptors in pituitary gland causing LH levels to drop 2 days after drug administration.
  - Rapid drop in testosterone production occurs.
  - Absence of flare due to lack of testosterone level increase after drug administration
  - May be useful in patients unable to tolerate an increase in disease-related symptoms that would accompany a testosterone level increase and disease flare
  - Administered by injection (see **Table 12–3**)

Surgical Castration[26]

- Bilateral orchiectomy removes testicular androgens.

Advantage
- Minimal risk
- Rapid reduction in testosterone level

TABLE 12–3 LHRH Agonists

Drug	Formulation	Dosage	Side Effects/Precautions
Abarelix (Plenaxis)	Injectable suspension Single-dose vial of sterile powder to be reconstituted with 0.9% sodium chloride, USP	100 mg IM to buttock on day 1, 15, 29, and q 4 weeks thereafter	Systemic allergic reactions have occurred—patients should be observed in office at least 30 minutes after each injection May elevate transaminase levels—monitor LFTs May prolong QT interval Decreased effectiveness in patients > 225 lbs
	Must be administered within 24 hrs of reconstitution	Effectiveness beyond 12 months has not been established	Decreased effectiveness with prolonged use—monitor serum testosterone levels on day 29 and q 8 weeks thereafter

Product information, Praecis Pharmaceuticals, Inc. 2003.
Source: Stempkowski L. Hormonal therapy. In: Held-Warmkessel, J., ed. *Contemporary Issues in Prostate Cancer: A Nursing Perspective* (2nd ed). Jones and Bartlett Publishers, 2006, 248–283. Reprinted with permission by Jones and Bartlett Publishers.

- Cost-effective
- Permanent
- No need for injections

Disadvantages
- Irreversible
- Eliminates option of using other hormonal therapies in clinical trials
- May not be appropriate for men concerned about body image
- Requires surgery

Pure Antiandrogens (see Table 12–4)
- Nonsteroidal antiandrogens
- Bind to AR in prostate and block AR
- No impact on circulating levels of testosterone

Side effects
- Breast tenderness
- Gynecomastia—probably due to altered estrogen balance and increased level of estradiol
- Hot flashes
- Anemia
- Asthenia
- Liver dysfunction—monitor liver function tests before start of therapy, at 1 month, and then every 3 months. Drug is to be stopped with development of hepatotoxicity (increased liver function tests or other signs of impaired liver function)
  - Cholestatic jaundice
  - Hepatic necrosis
  - Hepatic encephalopathy

TABLE 12–4 Pure Antiandrogens

Drug	Dosage	Financial Assistance
Flutamide/Eulexin	750 mg/day 125 mg capsules, 2 capsules q 8 hrs	Commitment to Care Ph: 1-800-521-7157
Bilcalutamide/Casodex	50 mg qd	Financial Assistance Program Ph: 1-800-424-3727
Nilatutamide Nilandron/Anandron	1st month: 300 mg/day, 50 mg tabs, 6 tabs/day Maintenance: 150 mg/day, 50 mg tabs, 3 tabs/day	Financial Assistance Program Ph: 1-800-221-4025

Product Information, Schering Corporation, 1996.
Product Information, Zeneca Pharmaceuticals, 1995.
Product Information, Hoechst Marion Roussel, 1996.
Source: Stempkowski L. Hormonal therapy. In: Held-Warmkessel, J., ed. *Contemporary Issues in Prostate Cancer: A Nursing Perspective* (2nd ed). Jones and Bartlett Publishers, 2006, 248–283. Reprinted with permission by Jones and Bartlett Publishers.

Drug-Specific Side Effects

- Flutamide—diarrhea. Manage with antidiarrheals or bulk-forming agents
- Nilutamide
  - Reversible interstitial lung disease; symptoms—progressive exertional dyspnea, cough, chest pain, fever—managed by stopping drug. Educate patient to monitor for these symptoms and report them immediately.
  - Alcohol intolerance—patient education and safety instructions must be provided to the patient and family.
  - Visual disturbances/night vision changes—patient education and safety instructions must be provided to the patient and family.

Steroidal Antiandrogens[22]

- Inhibit LH and block AR
- Megestrol acetate is one drug used.

Side effects
- Sexual dysfunction
- Decreased libido
- Impotence
- Thrombotic events

Total Androgen Blockade (TAB)

- Combination therapy with orchiectomy or LHRH agonist plus an antiandrogen to maximize androgen suppression by blocking both adrenal and testicular androgens (see **Table 12–5**)

INDICATIONS FOR HORMONAL MANIPULATION[30-31]

Metastatic Prostate Cancer

- Hormonal therapy produces response in 80% of patients with symptomatic metastatic prostate cancer.

TABLE 12-5 Biochemical Effects of Primary Hormonal Therapy

Biochemical Effect	Therapy				
	Orchiectomy	LHRH Agonists	Pure Antiandrogens	Steroid Antiandrogens	Total Androgen Blockade*
Removes source of testosterone	Yes				
Inhibits LHRH secretion by the hypothalamus		Yes			Yes
Inhibits LH secretion by the pituitary		Yes		Yes	Yes
Blocks binding of DHT to androgen receptor			Yes	Yes	Yes

*Orchiectomy or LHRH agonist plus antiandrogen.
LHRH, luteinizing hormone-releasing hormone; LH, luteinizing; DHT, dihydrotestosterone.
Data compiled from Brufsky and Kantoff,[2] and Boccon-Gibod.[27]
Source: Stempkowski L. Hormonal therapy. In: Held-Warmkessel, J., ed. *Contemporary Issues in Prostate Cancer: A Nursing Perspective* (2nd ed). Jones and Bartlett Publishers, 2006, 248–283. Reprinted with permission by Jones and Bartlett Publishers.

- Impact on symptom reduction, including urinary obstruction, bone pain, appetite increases, and improved well-being
- Reduced prostate-specific antigen (PSA) level
- Reduced tumor size
- Routine use of TAB not recommended for first-line hormonal therapy

Neoadjuvant Hormonal Therapy

Before surgery[32, 33]
- To downstage tumor, additional research is required; not recommended for use outside clinical trial
- No evidence that disease-free survival affected
- Negative impact on QOL

Before radiation therapy[34–40]
- May have synergy
- Both produce apoptosis by different mechanisms of action
- May decrease local progression rates at 5 years
- Length of therapy with neoadjuvant hormonal therapy is not well defined. May be as short as 6 months or may be longer
- Beneficial for men receiving external beam therapy or brachytherapy
- Brachytherapy patients receiving preimplant androgen deprivation therapy may have reduced tumor size and better local control.

Adjuvant Therapy[2]

- May be useful in men at risk of disease recurrence and metastases—T3 disease, positive lymph nodes, local disease with high-risk features

- May delay time to progression and improve survival
- Risks versus benefits of early hormonal therapy need to be evaluated for the individual patient.

Postradical Prostatectomy Recurrence[26]

- Patients may be candidates for hormonal therapy if they
  - Are postradical prostatectomy with no evidence of disease and detectable PSA
  - Have detectable PSA and positive surgical margins
  - Have T3c disease
  - Rising PSA > 0.3ng/mL after radical prostatectomy with increasing levels on two or more assessments
  - May be administered alone or with radiation therapy

Postradiation Therapy Recurrence[41]

- Hormonal therapy may be indicated in patients after radiation therapy with a rising PSA or local recurrence after a workup.

Node Positive (D1) Disease[42–44]

- May be indicated in patients without metastases but with locally advanced disease
- More research needed to determine the best time to start therapy.
- Additional variables to be considered are drug side effects and the patient's life expectancy.

SIDE EFFECT MANAGEMENT

Patient Education

- Includes spouse, significant other
- Initiate while patient is considering types of hormonal therapy offered by physician
- Encourage participation in a support group to assist with adapting to treatment-related side effects

Hot Flashes[45–53]

- Common side effect
- Variable intensity and duration
- Due to vasomotor activity
- May not go away with time
- A number of agents are available that have been found to be helpful, but more research is needed
- See **Table 12–6** for management options.

Fatigue[16, 54, 55]

- Common side effect
- Affects quality of life (QOL)
- Onset delayed
- Etiology multifactorial—may be due to reduced testosterone levels, anemia, pain, poor nutrition, psychosocial issues, and other factors
- Interventions include patient education, exercise, maintaining fatigue diary, and changing to different medication in same drug class

Erectile Dysfunction[56, 57]

- Common effect of testosterone level reduction
- Impacts on QOL

TABLE 12–6 Treatment Options for Relief of Hot Flashes

Drug	Dosage	Potential Side Effects
Megestrol acetate (Megace)[46]	20 mg bid	Episodes of chills Appetite stimulation Weight gain Symptoms of carpal tunnel syndrome
Clonidine (Catapres)[49]	Transdermal 0.1 mg weekly	Hypotension Allergic skin reaction to transdermal preparation
Medroxyprogesterone acetate (Depo-Provera)	400 mg IM	None reported when used every 6 months or less often
Venlafaxine[51]	12.5 mg po bid	Well tolerated at low doses Nausea, diarrhea, loss of appetite have been reported
Transdermal estrogen[52]	0.05 mg to 0.10 mg	Well tolerated Mild breast swelling and nipple tenderness have been reported

Data compiled from Loprinzi et al.,[46] Quella et al.,[51] Parra and Gregory,[49] and Gerber et al.[52]

Source: Stempkowski L. Hormonal therapy. In: Held-Warmkessel, J., ed. *Contemporary Issues in Prostate Cancer: A Nursing Perspective* (2nd ed). Jones and Bartlett Publishers, 2006, 248–283. Reprinted with permission by Jones and Bartlett Publishers.

- Cause may be multifactorial
- Important considerations in patients considering hormonal therapy
- Testicular and penile atrophy may also occur
- See **Table 12–7** for treatment options.[56, 57]

Osteoporosis[17, 18, 20, 21, 58]

- Bone loss occurs with loss of androgens
- Side effect of LHRH agonists is reduced bone mineral density and risk of fractures
- Bone density loss is greatest the first 2 years of therapy and then the rate of loss decreases but persists.
- In men receiving LHRH agonist therapy, the rate of osteoporosis hip fractures is 5% (3x the rate of age-matched controls).[18]
- Management of men initiating hormonal therapy consists of obtaining bone mineral density studies at the beginning of therapy and periodically thereafter.
- Patients should be encouraged to exercise.
- Additional potential risk factors include smoking and being underweight.
- Research is needed on incidence, severity, and impact of exercise, lifestyle changes, and bisphosphonates on the management of osteoporosis
- See **Figure 12–1**.

HORMONE–REFRACTORY DISEASE—ANDROGEN INDEPENDENCE[2]

- Response to androgen-reduction therapy occurs in 80–90% of patients
- Etiology of loss of androgen response may be related to inherent heterogeneity of response of prostate cancer cells to androgens.

TABLE 12–7 Treatment Options for Men with Erectile Dysfunction

Treatment	Advantages	Disadvantages
External vacuum devices[56]	Inexpensive Can be used with other treatment options	Mechanical: requires preparation time Produces cool erection Side effects include bruising, discomfort.
5 Phosphodiesterase Inhibitors Sildenafil (Viagra)[57]	Oral tablets	Side effects include headache, flushing, dyspepsia, nasal congestion, visual changes. Concurrent use of nitrates absolutely contraindicated. Concurrent use of alpha-blockers not recommended.
Vardenafil (Levitra)	Selective 5 phosphodiesterase inhibitor and consequently not as likely to cause visual changes	
Tadalafil (Cialis)	Reports of effectiveness as long as 36 hrs after taking Concurrent use of alpha-blocker, Flomax, not contraindicated	In addition to above side effects, muscle aches and back pain may be experienced, usually resolving in 48 hrs
Alprostadil (MUSE) urethral suppository	Minimally invasive Produces rapid natural-appearing erection	Requires test dose Potential urethral burning discomfort Potential for priapism Not effective with severe blood flow problem
Alprostadil penile injection therapy[56] (Caverject, Edex)		Requires test dose Potential urethral burning, discomfort, priapism, fibrosis Not effective with severe blood flow problem
Implantable penile prosthesis[56]	Use as directed No preparation time Increases girth of penis	Expensive Requires surgical procedure Risk of infection, erosion of device, device failure

Product information, Bayer Pharmaceuticals, 2003.
Product information, Lilly ICOS, 2004.
Product information, Vivus Inc, 1996.
Source: Stempkowski L. Hormonal therapy. In: Held-Warmkessel, J., ed. *Contemporary Issues in Prostate Cancer: A Nursing Perspective* (2nd ed). Jones and Bartlett Publishers, 2006, 248–283. Reprinted with permission by Jones and Bartlett Publishers.

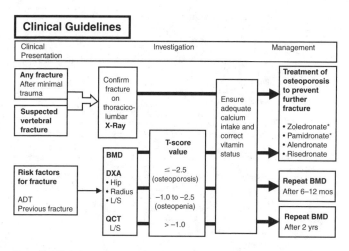

Clinical Guidelines

Clinical Presentation	Investigation	Management

Figure 12-1 Clinical guidelines

A clinical algorithm for identifying and managing high-risk men with prostate carcinoma who are beginning to receive or are receiving androgen deprivation therapy (ADT). Asterisks indicate agents that do not currently have approval from the United States Food and Drug Administration for use in the treatment of osteoporosis.

BMD: bone mineral density; DXA: dual-energy x-ray absorptiometry; L/S: lumbar spine; QCT: quantitative computed tomography.

Reprinted with permission of Wiley-Liss, Inc., a subsidiary of John Wiley & Sons, Inc.

Source: Diamond TH, Higano CS, Smith MR, et al. Osteoporosis in men with prostate carcinoma receiving androgen-deprivation therapy: recommendations for diagnosis and therapies. *Cancer* 2004; 100: 892–898.

Androgen Withdrawal Response[2, 59–64]

- Primary salvage therapy after demonstration of disease progression while receiving antiandrogen therapy is to stop antiandrogen therapy. Approximately 25% of patients will respond.
- After prolonged exposure to antiandrogens, cancer cells may become dependent on drug for growth.
- Drug removal may result in cancer cell regression with reduced PSA levels.
- Time to response of antiandrogen withdrawal (flutamide withdrawal syndrome) varies based on the half-life of the antiandrogen used.

Secondary Hormonal Manipulation[26, 59, 62, 65–69]

- Used after withdrawal of antiandrogens
- LHRH agent is continued for the life of patient to maintain testicular androgen suppression and present disease flare.
- Trial of a different antiandrogen. Patients who are asymptomatic and have a low burden of disease and responded to one antiandrogen are more likely to respond to a different one.[59]

- Response rates are low; duration of effect is short
- Corticosteroids—response rate is 20–25%
- Ketoconazole—response rate is 20–30%
  - Dose: 200–400 mg tid
  - Side effects include nausea, vomiting, rash, nail changes, edema, gynecomastia, and hepatotoxicity.
  - Administered with hydrocortisone
- Aminoglutethimide—response rate is 0–49%
  - Dose: 1000–1750 mg/day
  - Side effects include lethargy, nausea, rash, edema, hypothyroidism, and increased levels on liver function tests.
  - Patient must receive glucocorticoid replacement therapy with hydrocortisone while receiving aminoglutethimide.
- Diethylstilbestrol (DES)—response rate is 15–20%
  - Dose: 1–3 mg/day
  - Side effects include thrombotic events, nausea, vomiting, fluid retention, gynecomastia, mastodynia, and increased levels on liver function tests.
- Progestins
  - Medroxyprogesterone—reduces bone pain. Dose: 500–1200 mg/day; side effects include edema and cardiovascular events
  - Megestrol acetate—little activity
  - See **Table 12-8**.

Clinical trials of new hormonal agents may be an option.
- Chemotherapy—see Chapter 13

NEW APPROACHES TO HORMONAL MANIPULATION/ INVESTIGATIONAL THERAPIES

Peripheral Androgen Blockade[70, 71]

- Use of 5α-reductase inhibitor (finasteride) plus antiandrogen
- Blocks testosterone conversion and AR binding
- Does not reduce testosterone levels, and may reduce side effects associated with androgen deprivation therapy.
- May prolong time to progression with few side effects
- More research is needed.

Intermittent Androgen Suppression[71–74]

- TAB administered in intermittent manner until there is evidence of androgen independence
  - While off therapy, patients may experience increased potency and libido.
  - Initial TAB therapy may last 9–12 months followed by 6–9 months off therapy.
- TAB not administered in this manner may not affect survival.
- Used in stage D2 disease, disease relapse after radiation therapy, or radical prostatectomy
- Currently in phase III clinical trials.

Monotherapy[2, 75–78]

- Use of pure antiandrogen only; serum testosterone levels are not affected
- A number of clinical trials have been completed comparing antiandrogen monotherapy with a control arm of placebo or castration.
- Additional clinical trials are needed.

TABLE 12–8 Biochemical Effects of Secondary Hormonal Manipulation

Biochemical Effect	DES	Ketoconazole	Aminoglutethimide	Progestins	Corticosteroids
Inhibits 5-α-reductase				Yes	
Inhibits LH secretion by pituitary	Yes				
Inhibits LHRH secretoin by the hypothalamus	Yes			Yes	
Inhibits production of ACTH with resulting decrease in adrenal steroid production					Yes
Inhibits cytochrome P-450-mediated adrenal androgenesis		Yes	Yes	Yes	
Inhibits testicular androgenesis	Yes	Yes			
Blocks binding of DHT to androgen receptor				Yes	

DES, Diethylstilbestrol; LH, luteinizing hormone; LHRH, LH-releasing hormone, ACTH, corticotropin; DHT, dihydrotestosterone.
Data compiled from Brufsky and Kantoff,[2] Small and Srinivas,[62] and Small et al.[64]
Source: Stempkowski L. Hormonal therapy. In: Held-Warmkessel, J., ed. *Contemporary Issues in Prostate Cancer: A Nursing Perspective* (2nd ed). Jones and Bartlett Publishers, 2006, 248–283. Reprinted with permission by Jones and Bartlett Publishers.

References

1. McLeod DG, Crawford ED, DeAntoni EP. Combined androgen blockade: the gold standard for metastatic prostate cancer. *Eur Urol.* 1997;32(suppl 3):70–77.
2. Brufsky A, Kantoff PW. Hormonal therapy for prostate cancer. In: Ernstoff MS, Heaney JA, Peschel RE, eds. *Urol Cancer.* Cambridge, Mass: Blackwell Science; 1997:160–180.
3. Anderson KM, Laio S. Selective retention of dihydrotestosterone by prostatic cell nuclei. *Nature.* 1968;219:277–278.
4. Veldscholte J, Berrevoets CA, Zegers ND, et al. Hormone-induced dissociation of the androgen receptor-heat-shock protein complex: use of a new monoclonal antibody to distinguish transformed from nontransformed receptors. *Biochemistry.* 1992;31:7422–7430.

5. Davies P, Rushmere NK. Association of glucocorticoid receptors with prostate nuclear sites for androgen receptors and with androgen response elements. *J Mol Endocrinol.* 1990;5:117–127.

6. Labrie F. Intracrinology. *Mol Cell Endocrinol.* 1991;78:C113–C118.

7. Geller J. Basis for hormonal management of advanced prostatic cancer. *Cancer.* 1993;71:1039–1045.

8. Baird DT, Uno A, Melbe JC. Adrenal secretion of androgens and estrogens. *J Endocrinol.* 1969;45:135–136.

9. Harper ME, Pike A, Peeling WB, et al. Steroids of adrenal origin metabolized by human prostatic tissue both in vivo and in vitro. *J Endocrinol.* 1974;60:117–125.

10. Labrie F, Belanger A, Simard J, et al. Combination therapy for prostate cancer: Endocrine and biologic basis of its choice as new standard first-line therapy. *Cancer.* 1993;71:1059–1067.

11. Lachance Y, Luu-The V, Labrie C, et al. Characterization of human 3-beta hydroxysteroid dehydrogenase/delta-5 isomerase gene and its expression in mammalian cells. *J Biol Chem.* 1990;265:20469–20475.

12. Briehl MM, Miesfeld RL. Isolation and characterization of transcripts induced by androgen withdrawal and apoptotic cell death in the rat ventral prostate. *Mol Endocrinol.* 1991;5:1381–1388.

13. Kyprianou N, Martikainen P, Davis L, et al. Programmed cell death as a new target for prostate cancer therapy. *Cancer Surg.* 1991;11:265–277.

14. Martikainen P, Kyprianou N, Tucker RW, et al. Programmed death of nonproliferating androgen-independent prostate cancer cells. *Cancer Res.* 1991;51:4693–4700.

15. Harris MG, Coleman SG, Faulds D, Chrisp P. Nilutamide: a review of its pharmacodynamic and pharmacokinetic properties, and therapeutic efficacy in prostate cancer. *Drugs & Aging.* 1993;3:9–25.

16. Portenoy RK, Miaskowski C. Assessment and management of cancer-related fatigue. In: Berger AM, Portenoy RK, Weissman DE, eds. *Principles and Practice of Supportive Oncology.* Philadelphia, Pa: Lippincott-Raven; 1998:109–118.

17. Stepan JJ, Lachman M, Zverina J, et al. Castrated men exhibit bone loss: effect of calcitonin treatment on biochemical indices of bone remodeling. *J Clin Endocrinol Metab.* 1989;69:523–527.

18. Townsend MF, Sanders WH, Northway RO, Graham SD Jr. Bone fractures associated with luteinizing hormone-releasing hormone agonists used in the treatment of prostate carcinoma. *Cancer.* 1997;79:545–550.

19. Sisson de Castro JA. Alendronate treatment of osteoporosis in men: short-term bone mass response. *J Bone Miner Res.* 1995;11(suppl 1):341.

20. Daniell HW. Osteoporosis after orchiectomy for prostate cancer. *J Urol.* 1997;157:439–444.

21. Diamond TH, Higano CS, Smith MR, Guise TA, Singer FR. Osteoporosis in men with prostate cancer receiving androgen-deprivation therapy: recommendations for diagnosis and therapies. *Cancer.* 2004;100:892–898.

22. Bubley, GJ. Is the flare phenomenon clinically significant? *Urology.* 2001;58(suppl 2A):5–9.

23. Labrie F, Dupont A, Belanger A, Lachance R. Flutamide eliminates the risk of disease flare in prostatic cancer patients treated with luteinizing hormone-releasing hormone agonist. *J Urol.* 1987;138:804–806.

24. McLeod D, Zinner N, Tomera K, et al. A phase 3, multicenter, open-label, randomized study of aberelix versus leuprolide acetate in men with prostate cancer. *Urology.* 2001;58:756–761.

25. Weckermann D, Harzmann R. Hormone therapy in prostate cancer: LHRH antagonists versus LHRH analogues. *Eur Urol.* 2004;46:279–283.
26. Prostate cancer guideline. June 2004. *The Complete Library of NCCN Clinical Practice Guidelines in Oncology (CD-ROM).* Jenkintown, Pa: National Comprehensive Cancer Network.
27. Boccon-Gibod L. Quoted in: Crawford ED. The role of antiandrogens in hormonal therapy: Part 1. Recorded symposium of the Societe Internationale d'Urologie, September 1997. *Comtemp Urol.* June 1998;43–57.
28. Blackledge G. Clinical progress with a new antiandrogen, Casodex (bicalutamide). *Eur Urol.* 1996;29(Suppl 2):96–104.
29. Bennett CL. Quoted in: Crawford ED. The role of antiandrogens in hormonal therapy: Part 1. Recorded symposium of the Societe Internationale d'Urologie, September 1997. *Comtemp Urol.* June 1998;43–57.
30. Resnick, MI. Hormonal therapy in prostatic cancer. *Urology.* 1984;24:18–23.
31. Laufer M, Denmeade SR, Sinibaldi VJ, et al. Complete androgen blockade for prostate cancer: What went wrong? *J Urol.* 2000;164:3–9.
32. Chun J, Pruthi RS. Is neoadjuvant hormonal therapy before radical prostatectomy indicated? *Urol Int.* 2004;72:275–80.
33. Namiki S, Saito S, Tochigi T, et al. Impact of hormonal therapy prior to radical prostatectomy on the recovery of quality of life. *Int J Urol.* 2005;12:173–181.
34. Roach M. Neoadjuvant therapy prior to radiotherapy for clinically localized prostate cancer. *Eur Urol.* 1997;32(suppl 3):48–54.
35. Pilepich MV, Sause WT, Shipley WU, et al. Androgen deprivation with radiation therapy compared with radiation therapy alone for locally advanced prostate carcinoma: a randomized comparative trial of the Radiation Therapy Oncology Group. *Urology.* 1995;45:616–623.
36. Hanks GE, Pajak TF, Porter A, et al. Phase III trial of long-term adjuvant androgen deprivation after neoadjuvant hormonal cytoreduction and radiotherapy in locally advanced carcinoma of the prostate: the Radiation Oncology Group Protocol 92–02. *J Clin Oncol.* 2004;22:386.
37. Bolla M, Collette L, Blank L, et al. Long-term results with immediate androgen suppression and external irradiation in patients with locally advanced prostate cancer (an EORTC study), a phase III randomized. *Lancet.* 2002;360:103–106.
38. D'Amico AV, Manola J, Loffredo M, et al. 6-month androgen suppression plus radiation therapy vs. radiation therapy alone for patients with clinically localized prostate cancer. *JAMA.* 2004;292:821–827.
39. Stock RG, Stone NN. The effect of prognostic factors on therapeutic outcome following transperineal prostate brachytherapy. *Semin Surg Oncol.* 1997;13:454–460.
40. Stone NN, Stock RG. Neoadjuvant hormonal therapy improves the outcomes of patients undergoing radioactive seed implantation for localized prostate cancer. *Mol Urol.* 1999;3:239–244.
41. Cox JD, Gallagher MJ, Hammond EH et al. Consensus statements on radiation therapy of prostate cancer: guidelines for prostate re-biopsy after radiation and for radiation therapy with rising PSA levels after radical prostatectomy. American Society for Therapeutic Radiology and Oncology (ASTRO) Consensus Panel. *J Clin Oncol.* 1999;17:1155.
42. Van Aubel OG, Hoekstra W, Schroder FH. Early orchiectomy for patients with stage D1 prostate cancer. *J Urol.* 1985;134:292–294.
43. Kramolowsky E. The value of testosterone deprivation in stage D1 carcinoma of the prostate. *J Urol.* 1988;139:1242–1244.

44. Messing EM, Manola J, Sarosdy M, et al. Immediate hormonal therapy compared with observation after radical prostatectomy and pelvic lymphadenectomy in men with node-positive prostate cancer. *N Engl J Med.* 1999;341:1781–1788.
45. Karling P, Hammar M, Varenhorst E. Prevalence and duration of hot flushes after surgical or medical castration in men with prostatic carcinoma. *J Urol.* 1994;152: 1170–1173.
46. Loprinzi CL, Michalak JC, Quella SK, et al. Megestrol acetate for the prevention of hot flashes. *N Engl J Med.* 1994;331:347–352.
47. Quella SK, Loprinzi CL, Sloan JA, et al. Long-term use of megestrol acetate by cancer survivors for the treatment of hot flashes. *Cancer.* 1998;82:1784–1788.
48. Bressler LR, Murphy CM, Shevrin DH, Warren RF. Use of clonidine to treat hot flashes secondary to leuprolide or goserelin. *Ann Pharmacother.* 1993;27:182–185.
49. Parra RO, Gregory JG. Treatment of post-orchiectomy hot flashes with transdermal administration of clonidine. *J Urol.* 1990;143:753.
50. Brosman SA. Depo-Provera as a treatment for "hot flashes" in men on androgen ablation therapy. Proceedings of the 90th annual meeting of the American Urological Association. [Abstract 877] *J Urol.* 1995;153:448A.
51. Quella SK, Loprinzi CL, Sloan J, et al. Pilot evaluation of venlafaxine for the treatment of hot flashes in men undergoing androgen ablation therapy for prostate cancer. *J Urol.* 1999;162:98–102.
52. Gerber GS, Zagaja GP, Ray PS, Rukstalis DB. Transdermal estrogen in the treatment of hot flushes in men with prostate cancer. *Urology.* 2000;55:97–101.
53. Jeffery SM, Pepe JJ, Popovich LM, Vitagliano G. Gabapentin for hot flashes in prostate cancer. *Ann Pharmacother.* 2002;26:433–436.
54. Stone P, Hardy J, Huddart R, et al. Fatigue in patients with prostate cancer receiving hormonal therapy. *Eur J Cancer.* 2000;36:1134.
55. Segal RJ, Reid RD, Courneya KS, et al. Resistance exercise in men receiving androgen deprivation therapy for prostate cancer. *J Clin Oncol.* 2003;21:1653.
56. Bryant R, Boarini J. Treatment options for men with sexual dysfunction. *J ET Nurs.* 1992;19:131–142.
57. Goldstein I, Lue TF, Padma-Nathan H, et al. Oral sildenafil in the treatment of erectile dysfunction. *N Engl J Med.* 1998;338:1397–1404.
58. Smith MR, Eastham J, Gleason DM, et al. Randomized controlled trial of zoledronic acid to prevent bone loss in men receiving androgen deprivation therapy for non-metastatic prostate cancer. *J Urol.* 2003;169:2008–2012.
59. Ryan CJ, Small EJ. Role of secondary hormonal therapy in the management of recurrent prostate cancer. *Urology.* 2003;62(suppl 6B):87–94.
60. Herrada J, Dieringer P, Logothetis CJ. Characteristics of patients with androgen-independent prostatic carcinoma whose serum prostate specific antigen decreased following flutamide withdrawal. *J Urol.* 1996;155:620–623.
61. Figg WD, Sartor O, Cooper MR, et al. Prostate specific antigen decline following the discontinuation of flutamide in patients with stage D2 prostate cancer. *Am J Med.* 1995;98:412–414.
62. Small EJ, Srinivas S. The antiandrogen withdrawal syndrome. *Cancer.* 1995;76: 1428–1434.
63. Scher HI, Zhang ZF, Nanus D, Kelly WK. Hormone and antihormone withdrawal: Implications for the management of androgen-independent prostate cancer. *Urology.* 1996;47:61–69.

64. Small EJ, Schellhammer P, Venner G, et al. A double-blind assessment of anti-androgen withdrawal from casodex or eulexin therapy while continuing luteinizing hormone releasing hormone analogue therapy for patients with stage D2 prostate cancer [abstract]. *Proc Am Soc Clin Oncol.* 1996;15:255.

65. Smith DC. Secondary hormonal therapy. *Semin Urol Oncol.* 1997;15:3–12.

66. Small EJ, Baron AD, Fippin L, Apodaca D. Ketoconazole retains activity in advanced prostate cancer patients with progression despite flutamide withdrawal. *J Urol.* 1997;157:1204–1207.

67. Johansson JE, Andersson SO, Holmberg L. High-dose medroxyprogesterone acetate vs. estramustine in therapy-resistant prostate cancer. *Br J Urol.* 1991;68:67–73.

68. Sasagawa I, Satomi S. Effect of high-dose medroxyprogesterone acetate on plasma hormone levels and pain relief in patients with advanced prostate cancer. *Br J Urol.* 1990;65:278–281.

69. Bezwoda WR. Treatment of stage D2 prostate cancer refractory to or relapsed following castration plus estrogens. *Br J Urol.* 190;66:196–201.

70. Ornstein DK, Rao GS, Johnson B, Charlton ET, Andriole GL. Combined finasteride and flutamide therapy in men with advanced prostate cancer. *Urology.* 1996;48:901–905.

71. Trachtenberg J. Innovative approaches to the hormonal treatment of advanced prostate cancer. *Eur Urol.* 1997;32(suppl 3):78–80.

72. Goldenberg SL, Bruchronsky N, Gleave ME, et al. Intermittent androgen suppression in the treatment of prostate cancer: a preliminary report. *Urology.* 1995;47:956–961.

73. Rashid MH, Chaudhary UB. Intermittent androgen deprivation therapy for prostate cancer. *Oncologist.* 2004;9:295–301.

74. Tunn U, Eckart O, Kienle E et al. Can intermittent androgen deprivation be an alternative to continuous androgen withdrawal in patients with PSA relapse? First results of the randomized prospective phase III clinical trial EC 507. *J Urol.* 2003;169(suppl 4):1481a.

75. Iversen P, Tyrrell CJ, Kaisary AV, et al. Bicalutamide monotherapy compared with castration in patients with nonmetastatic locally advanced prostate cancer: 6.3 years of follow-up. *J Urol.* 2000;164:1579–1582.

76. Tyrrell CJ, Kaisary AV, Iversen P, et al. A randomized comparison of Casodex (bicalutamide) 150 mg monotherapy versus castration in the treatment of metastatic and locally advanced prostate cancer. *Eur Urol.* 1998;33:447–456.

77. Fourcade RO, Chatelain C, Poterre M. An open multicenter randomized study to compare the effect and safety of Casodex (bicalutamide) 150 mg monotherapy with castration plus nilutamide in metastatic prostate cancer [abstract]. *Eur Urol.* 1998;33(suppl 1):88 Abs 349.

78. See WA, Wirth MP, McLeod DG, et al. Bicalutamide as immediate therapy either alone or as adjuvant to standard care of patients with localized or locally advanced prostate cancer: first analysis of the Early Prostate Cancer Program. *J Urol.* 2002;168: 429–435.

Treatment of Hormone-Refractory Prostate Cancer with Chemotherapy

INTRODUCTION

- Hormone-refractory prostate cancer (HRPC) is a type of prostate cancer that may be treated with chemotherapy.
- Median survival of patients is 15 to 16 months.[1, 2] Median survival in patients with PSA only elevation may be longer.
- Traditionally, patients responded poorly to chemotherapy.
- Only recently has docetaxel-based chemotherapy demonstrated a survival advantage.[3, 4]

Challenges in Treating HRPC

- Elderly population of patients with other health problems
- Poor bone marrow reserve related to bone marrow metastases or prior radiation therapy to bone marrow[5]

Disease Progression Characterized By[6, 7]

- Prostate-specific antigen (PSA) increase
- Increased disease on diagnostic studies: bone scan, magnetic resonance imaging (MRI), computed tomography (CT) scan
- Worsening symptoms, such as pain, urinary obstruction, anemia, weight loss, bladder outlet obstruction, and fatigue

PUPROSES OF CHEMOTHERAPY

- Palliation of symptoms
- Potential for increased survival

CHEMOTHERAPY CANDIDATES

Potential Candidates for Therapy Include patients with the Following Factors

- Need for disease palliation
- Presence of painful metastases or other symptoms reducing quality of life
- Hormone therapy resistance with documented disease progression and hormonal insensitivity[8, 9]
- Factors important in the decision to initiate chemotherapy include tumor growth rate, extent of disease, symptoms, medical condition, comorbid diseases, and patient willingness to undergo therapy. Treatment may produce side effects and unknown benefit.
- Research trial candidates must meet eligibility criteria and have none of the ineligibility criteria.

- Hormone manipulation is continued to block testosterone even in presence of HRPC.[9]

Potential Benefits of Therapy

- Disease palliation, reduced pain, reduced need for analgesics, improved quality of life, and potential for increased survival

Patient Education Is Crucial at the Initiation of Therapy and During Therapy

- Education includes drugs: route of administration, side effects, treatment plan, and self-care measures. Use both oral and written educational formats and reinforce education during each treatment session

---

CHEMOTHERAPY

Single-Agent Chemotherapy

- Drugs listed in **Table 13–1**[10–17] have been investigated for their usefulness in treating HRPC.
- Side effects vary based on the regimen used.

Side Effects

- Myelosuppression (anemia, neutropenia, thrombocytopenia)
- Allergic reactions
- Gastrointestinal disturbances—anorexia, nausea, vomiting, diarrhea, mucositis
- Fatigue
- Alopecia
- Peripheral edema
- Gynecomastia
- Cardiac and cardiovascular toxicities
- Skin and nail changes
- Ocular toxicities
- Urine color changes
- Steroid-induced hyperglycemia
- Altered fluid and electrolyte balance
- Peripheral neuropathy
- Side effects vary in severity from mild or bothersome to severe and potentially life threatening.

Agents Used

- Mitoxantrone—anthracenedione antineoplastic agent related to doxorubicin, FDA-approved to treat HRPC
- Estramustine—compound product of nornitrogen mustard and estradiol, antimitotic agent; myelosuppression is rare when used as a single agent, FDA-approved to treat HRPC.
- Cyclophosphamide—alkylating agent; available in oral and intravenous formulations
- Paclitaxel (taxane)—antimicrotubule activity; treatment with this agent requires premedication with dexamethasone, diphenhydramine, intravenously (IV) plus cimetidine or another histamine-2 blocker. Must be administered through a 0.2 micron in-line filter through nonpolyvinyl chloride tubing with a glass, polypropylene, or other nonplasticized container. Hypersensitivity reactions may occur—routine patient monitoring of vital signs for bradycardia and hypotension is required.

TABLE 13–1 Single-Agent Chemotherapy Used in the Treatment of Prostate Cancer

Study	N	Major End Points	Treatment-Doses Administered
Raghavan et al.[10]	50	Measurable disease Symptoms	Mitoxantrone, IV 12–14 mg/m^2 q 21 days, no steroids
Iversen et al.[11]	129	Clinical progression • Death Adverse events • PSA Subjective response	280 mg estramustine po bid (daily total 560 mg) vs. placebo
Roth et al.[12]	21 evaluable	Measurable disease	Paclitaxel, IV by continuous infusion 135–170 mg/m^2 q 21 days
Hussain et al.[13]	22	Measurable disease PSA	VP-16 po 50 mg/m^2/day for 21 days, repeated q 28 days
Kojima et al.[14]	10, 9 were evaluable	> 50% PSA reduction, objective tumor response	Docetaxel 30 mg/m^2 IV weekly × 3 weeks followed by 2 weeks off
Schultz et al.[15]	21 evaluable	PSA	Docetaxel, 75 mg/m^2 q 21 days
Trivedi et al.[16]	18	≥ 50% reduction in PSA	150 mg/m^2 IV paclitaxel administered over 1 hour weekly for 6 weeks followed by 2 weeks off therapy
Raghaven et al.[17]	30	Symptom reduction Survival	Cyclophosphamide, 100 mg/m^2/day for 14 days, repeated q 28 days; dose reduced to 100 mg/day for patients with prior pelvic radiation therapy

Major Findings	Major Toxicities
Disease stabilization, 52%; reduced pain, 38%; reduced symptoms, 46%; no CRs, no PRs; median survival, 10 months	Myelosuppression Nail thickening Subungual hematomas
Median survival: placebo, 6.1 months; estramustine, 9.4 months; P=ns Subjective response: placebo, 7%; estramustine, 18%; P=ns	Breast tenderness Gynecomastia Diarrhea
Median survival, 9 months; 1 PR; 4 stable disease with PSA reductions of 16–24%; 11 stable disease	Leukopenia • Granulocytopenic fever • Cardiovascular events, including two deaths • Rash
2 PRs; minimally active drug; median survival, 31 weeks	Anemia • Granulocytopenia • Thrombocytopenia
5 patients with > 50% reduction in PSA and 4 of those 5 patients had > 75% PSA reduction. Two of these patients had a PR; 3 of these patients had reduced narcotic requirements.	Neutropenia Anemia
Median survival = 6 months PRs, 24%	Fatigue • Stomatitis • Small bowel obstruction • Gluteal abscess • Death from lung toxicity—pneumonia, pulmonary embolus in two patients • Neutropenia • Anemia • Mild edema • Anorexia • Myalgia • Alopecia • Steroid-induced hyperglycemia
1 CR + 3 PRs. 39% of patients had a ≥ 50% reduction in PSA	Peripheral neuropathy
Median survival from onset of treatment, 12.7 months; symptom reduction, 60%	Nausea • Vomiting • Anemia • Myelosuppression

IV, intravenous; PSA, prostate-specific antigen; NS, not significant; CI, continuous infusion; bid, twice daily.
Source: Held-Warmkessel, J. Treatment of hormone-refractory prostate cancer with chemotherapy. In: Held-Warmkessel, J., ed. *Contemporary Issues in Prostate Cancer: A Nursing Perspective* (2nd ed). Jones and Bartlett Publishers, 2006, 284–317. Reprinted with permission by Jones and Bartlett Publishers.

- Docetaxel (taxane)antimicrotubule activity. Premedications are required to reduce incidence of fluid retention. Hypersensitivity reactions may occur. FDA approved for treatment of HRPC.[4]
- Etoposide (VP-16)—inhibits topoisomerase II; allergic reactions may occur.
- Prednisone—single-agent, low-dose

CHEMOTHERAPY AND PREDNISONE

Mitoxantrone and Prednisone

- Food and Drug Administration (FDA) approved for the palliative treatment of HRPC. Multiple clinical trials have been completed (see **Table 13–2**).[18–24] In responding patients, symptoms were reduced; however, survival was not affected.[18, 20]
- Additional drugs have been added or the dose of mitoxantrone has been escalated in attempts to improve on outcome.

Estramustine and Docetaxel

- Multiple clinical trials have been done using these agents together (see **Table 13–3**).[21–32]
- Reduces PSA values[28–32]
- Additional drugs have been added to docetaxel-based regimens with the goal of improving outcomes, but more clinical trials are needed.

PHASE III STUDIES

- Studies compared the most effective agents: estramustine, docetaxel and dexamethasone with mitoxantrone and prednisone or prednisone and mitoxantrone with prednisone and docetaxel (see **Table 13–4**).[3–4]
- In the clinical trials, the docetaxel-based therapies produced better outcomes in terms of survival, reduced mortality, reduced PSA, reduced pain, and better

TABLE 13–2 Mitoxantrone-Based Studies

Study	N	Major End Points	Treatment-Doses Administered
Moore et al.[18]	27	Palliative response: pain, quality of life	Mitoxantrone, 12 mg/m^2 IV q 21 days with dose escalation by 2 mg/m^2 if nadir ANC > 1.0 × 10^9/L and platelets > 50 × 10^9/L at nadir, plus prednisone, 5 mg bid
Tannock et al.[19]	161 phase III	Pain relief, reduced analgesic scores	Mitoxantrone, 12 mg/m^2 IV q 21 days + prednisone, 5 mg bid vs. prednisone, 5 mg bid alone

quality of life. These were the first studies to demonstrate the ability of docetaxel-based chemotherapy to improve survival in HRPC.[3–4] Docetaxel plus
prednisone is considered the standard of care.
- Docetaxel-based therapy produces more side effects than mitoxantrone-based
therapy.

TREATMENT OPTIONS AFTER CHEMOTHERAPY FAILURE
- Clinical trials
- Referrals to social service, hospice, home care, or pain management team
- For patients with a good performance status, a different chemotherapy regimen
may be offered.

NURSING MANAGEMENT
- Usual settings for nursing care—outpatient clinic, physician's office, or patient's
home
- Patient education includes self-care management of expected side effects and
when to call the physician or nurse. Begins with introduction of concept of
chemotherapy and continues with each patient contact. Crucial to the successful
treatment of the patient receiving chemotherapy.
- Encourage phone calls with questions or problems. Follow up patient treatment
with a phone call 1–2 days after treatment to assess for problems and side effects and continue patient education.
- Management of psychosocial issues in collaboration with social worker or hospice team
- Nursing management includes assessing, planning, intervening, and
evaluating the plan of care (see **Table 13–5**),[31, 33–40] and collaborating with the
physician in management of patient side effects and toxicities.

Major Findings	Major Toxicities
Palliative CR, 16%; palliative PR, 20%; stable disease, 41%; median survival, 5.7 months	Nausea, neutropenia, alopecia, anorexia, constipation
Mitoxantrone-prednisone responses, 29%; Prednisone alone, 12% (P = .01). Response duration: mitoxantrone-prednisone, 43 weeks; prednisone, 18 weeks (P < .0001). mitoxantrone-prednisone response, 38%; prednisone response, 21%; no effect on survival in either group	Nausea, vomiting, hair loss, neutropenic fever. Cardiac toxicity with cumulative doses of 116–214 mg/m^2 mitoxantrone

continues

TABLE 13–2 Mitoxantrone-Based Studies, continued

Study	N	Major End Points	Treatment-Doses Administered
Kantoff et al.[20]	242	Survival Quality of life	Hydrocortisone, 40 mg/day with or without mitoxantrone, 14 mg/m² q 21 days
Sheen et al.[21]	28	Survival	8 mg/m² IV mitoxantrone every 3 weeks + 10 mg oral prednisolone bid
Ernst et al.[22]	209	Palliation of pain and quality of life	Prednisone 5 mg bid daily + mitoxantrone 12 mg/m² IV every 3 weeks and clodronate 1500 mg IV or placebo of IV saline
Berry et al.[23]	120	Time to treatment failure in asymptomatic patients with progressive HRPC (the time between starting therapy and development of progressive disease)	Mitoxantrone 12 mg/m² IV every 3 weeks + 5 mg prednisone orally bid vs. 5 mg prednisone orally bid
DeConti, et al.[24]	14 evaluable	PSA Measurable disease Pain Quality of life	Mitoxantrone, 12 mg/m², plus paclitaxel, 175 mg/m² q 21 days GM-CSF until ANC 1500/ml

ANC, absolute neutrophil count; bid, twice daily; CR, complete response; PR, partial response; IV, intravenous; GM-CSF, granulocyte-macrophage colony-stimulating factor; po, orally.

Major Findings	Major Toxicities
Median survival not affected 12.3 months (mitoxantrone-hydrocortisone) vs. 12.6 months (hydrocortisone); pain level improved	Myelotoxicity
Median survival = 12 months PSA reduced in 15 patients (≥ 50%) including 9 patients with ≥ 80% reduction. Pain reduced in 5 of 16 patients. Improved performance status in 9 patients. Two of 12 patients with measurable disease had a PR	Neutropenia Anemia Vomiting
Palliative end points not affected by clodronate. Survival of 10.8 months in clodronate arm and 11.5 months in placebo arm	Myelosuppression Infection Cardiovascular Nausea/vomiting Headache Shortness of breath
Time to treatment failure—8.1 months in mitoxantrone/prednisone group and 4.1 months in prednisone alone group. No affect on survival	Myelosuppression Pulmonary Renal GI Sepsis Melanoma Asthenia
Median survival > 11 months; responses, > 50% improvement in PSA, 64%; pain, 77%	Anaphylaxis Myelotoxicity Neutropenic fever Neurotoxicity

Source: Held-Warmkessel, J. Treatment of hormone-refractory prostate cancer with chemotherapy. In: Held-Warmkessel, J., ed. *Contemporary Issues in Prostate Cancer: A Nursing Perspective* (2nd ed). Jones and Bartlett Publishers, 2006, 284–317. Reprinted with permission by Jones and Bartlett Publishers.

TABLE 13-3 Estramustine-Docetaxel Clinical Trials

Study	N	Major End Points	Treatment-Doses Administered	Major Findings	Major Toxicities
Petrylak et al.[25]	34 evaluable for toxicity, 33 evaluable for response	PSA	Estramustine, 280 mg po tid days 1–5 + docetaxel given at 4 dose levels on day 2; 40, 60, 70 or 80 mg/m² IV + dexamethasone 20 mg given 6 and 12 hours and 15 minutes before docetaxel repeated every 21 days	Overall PSA response, 63%; reduced analgesic requirements, 53%; measurable disease, 28% PR Recommended phase II dose is 60–70 mg/m² IV based on prior level of chemotherapy exposure	• Fluid retention • Transaminitis • Granulocytopenia • Neutropenic fever • Nausea	• Vomiting • Hyperbilirubinemia • CVA • DVT • Extravasation
Kreis et al.[26, 27]	17	PSA	Estramustine po 14 mg/kg daily for 21 days + docetaxel 40, 60, 70, or 80 mg/m² IV every 21 days + Dexamethasone 8 mg po bid × 5 days to prevent fluid retention	14 of 17 patients with PSA response Recommended phase II docetaxel dose is 70 mg/m² IV docetaxel every 3 weeks with estramustine 12mg/kg	• Leukopenia • Fatigue • Diarrhea • Anemia • Increased LFTs • Anorexia	• Stomatitis • Epigastric pain • Hyponatremia • Hypocalcemia • Hypophosphatemia • Thromboembolic events
Petrylak et al.[28]	18 evaluable	PSA	280 mg estramustine po days 1–5 tid + docetaxel 70 mg/m² IV on day 2 + dexamethasone 20 mg given 6 and 12 hours and 15 minutes before docetaxel Cycles repeated every 21 days	84% of patients had a ≥ 50% reduction in PSA	• Neutropenia • Neutropenic fever • Transaminitis	• Edema • Fatigue • Vascular events
Savarere, et al.[29]	46 evaluable	Response rate; PSA	Estramustine 10 mg/kg/day po with dose divided up and administered tid days 1–5 repeated every 21 days + docetaxel 70 mg/m² IV day 2 repeated every 21 days with dexamethasone 8 mg bid days 1–3 of each cycle +	In 24 patients with measurable disease, 3 CRs + 9 PRs for a 50% RR. In 44 patients with PSA responses, 68% with ≥ 50% PSA reduction and 57% with ≥ 75% PSA reduction. For all patients, 3 CRs and 22 PRs. Median survival = 20 months	• Neutropenia • Anemia • Thrombocytopenia • Hyperglycemia • Edema	• Fatigue • Infection • Increased alkaline phosphatase • Dyspnea • Thromboembolic events

Study	Patients	Endpoints	Regimen	Results	Toxicities
Copur, et al.[30]	30 heavily pretreated, elderly patients with poor PS	PSA; pain, PS	Dexamethasone 4 mg bid days 1–3 + docetaxel 35 mg/m² IV on day 2 + estramustine tid days 1–3 (first 4 doses were 420 mg and last 5 doses were 280 mg). Repeated every 21 days.	Median survival = 20 months. 76% of patients with ≥ 50% reduction in PSA including 56% with ≥ 75% reduction. Reduced pain and improved PS in 70%	• Edema • DVT • Myelosuppression • Nausea • Asthenia • Diarrhea
Sinibaldi, et al.[31]	42 patients; 40 evaluable	PSA	Docetaxel 70 mg/m² IV 12 hours after first dose of estramustine + estramustine 280 mg po every 6 hours × 5 doses + coumadin 2 mg po daily + Dexamethasone 8 mg bid days 1–3 for patients numbered 1–14. For the other patients, 20 mg po 12 hours and 6 hours prior to docetaxel cycles repeated every 21 days.	> 50% PSA reduction = 45%. 59% of patients with pain reduction Median survival = 13.5 months	• Hyperglycemia • Nail changes • Skin changes • CHF/atrial fibrillation • Fatigue • Myelosuppression • Neutropenic fever • Diarrhea
Eymard, et al.[32]	92 patients; Arm A = 48 Arm B = 44	PSA, safety, QOL	Arm A = docetaxel 70 mg/m² IV day 1 + estramustine 560 mg/day × 5 days beginning 1 day before docetaxel + warfarin 1 mg/day vs. Arm B = docetaxel 75 mg/m² IV. Both arms received corticosteroids. Cycles repeated every 3 weeks.	PSA > 50% reduction Arm A = 68% Arm B = 29% PSA > 75% reduction Arm A = 36% Arm B = 16%	• Allergic reactions • Febrile neutropenia • Pulmonary edema • Neutropenia • Anemia • Thrombophlebitis

PSA = prostate-specific antigen; tid = three times a day; PR = partial response; CVA = cerebrovascular accident; DVT = deep vein thrombosis; po = orally; CR = complete response; RR = response rate; PS = performance status; QOL = quality of life

Source: Held-Warmkessel, J. Treatment of hormone-refractory prostate cancer with chemotherapy. In: Held-Warmkessel, J., ed. *Contemporary Issues in Prostate Cancer: A Nursing Perspective* (2nd ed). Jones and Bartlett Publishers, 2006, 284–317. Reprinted with permission by Jones and Bartlett Publishers.

TABLE 13–4 Phase III Docetaxel-Based Clinical Trials

Study	N	Major End Points	Drugs, Doses, Route, and Frequency of Administration
Petrylak et al.[3]	674; 338 received docetaxel and estramustine; 336 received mitoxantrone and prednisone	Overall survival	Estramustine 280 mg tid (one hour before meals or two hours after) days 1–5 (anticoagulation prophylaxis initiated 2 years into study to include 2 mg warfarin daily + 325 mg aspirin daily) + docetaxel 60 mg/m^2 IV on day 2 + dexamethasone 20 mg tid beginning night before docetaxel for a total dose of 60 mg per cycle OR 12 mg/m^2 mitoxantrone on day 1 + prednisone 5 mg bid Doses of docetaxel and mitoxantrone were increased to 70 mg/m^2 IV or 14 mg/m^2 IV respectively if patients did not develop grade 3 or 4 toxicities in cycle 1. LHRH agonists were continued throughout therapy. Cycles were repeated every 21 days
Tannock et al.[4]	1006; 337 in mitoxantrone group; 335 in the every 3 weeks docetaxel group; 334 in the weekly docetaxel group	Overall survival Pain QOL	5 mg prednisone + mitoxantrone 12 mg/m^2 IV every 3 weeks OR docetaxel 75 mg/m^2 IV every 3 weeks OR docetaxel 30 mg/m^2 IV weekly × 5 weeks followed by 1 week off therapy. Androgen ablative therapy continued throughout therapy. Cross-over therapy permitted for nonresponders

tid = three times a day; bid = twice a day; LHRH = luteinizing-hormone releasing hormone; QOL = quality of life.
Source: Held-Warmkessel, J. Treatment of hormone-refractory prostate cancer with chemotherapy. In: Held-Warmkessel, J., ed. *Contemporary Issues in Prostate Cancer: A Nursing Perspective* (2nd ed). Jones and Bartlett Publishers, 2006, 284–317. Reprinted with permission by Jones and Bartlett Publishers.

Major Findings	Major Toxicities
Median overall survival was 17.5 months in the docetaxel/estramustine group and 15.6 months in the mitoxantrone/prednisone group ($P = .02$). Resulted in a 20% reduction in mortality in the docetaxel/ estramustine group.	Neutropenic fevers Nausea Vomiting Infection Metabolic Neurologic events Death Side effects more serious in the docetaxel/estramustine group
Median survival = 16.5 months in mitoxantrone group; 18.9 months in every 3 weeks docetaxel group; 17.4 months in weekly docetaxel group. The three groups had ≥ 50% reduction in PSA—32%, 45%, 48%; reduced pain—22%, 35%, 31%; better QOL—13%, 22%, 23%. Docetaxel-based therapy improved survival	Side effects more common in docetaxel groups Neutropenia Fatigue Nausea Vomiting Diarrhea Sepsis Cardiac

TABLE 13–5 Standard of Care: Chemotherapy for the Management of Hormone-Refractory Prostate Cancer

NURSING DIAGNOSIS: Knowledge deficit related to chemotherapy, its side effects, and self-care activities

OUTCOME: Pt will verbalize understanding of purpose of chemotherapy, side effects, and how to manage side effects at home.

NURSING INTERVENTIONS:

1. Assess pt/SO understanding of the purpose of chemotherapy, side effects, and self-care.

2. Educate pt/SO as to drug action, expected side effects, and management (appropriate for regimen): myelosuppression; anorexia, nausea, vomiting; diarrhea; changes in urine color; alopecia; mucositis; peripheral edema; neuropathy; altered LFTs; allergic reactions; fatigue; cardiac; cardiovascular; hemorrhagic cystitis; myalgia; steroid-induced hyperglycemia.

3. Educate pt as to s-s requiring nurse-physician notification: fever (T $\geq$ 100.5°F), chills, bleeding, vomiting, dehydration, profound fatigue, mucositis, leg swelling.

4. Encourage pt/SO to verbalize questions, concerns about treatment, side effects and self-care.

5. Provide pt/SO with printed education materials to use as reference at home.

NURSING DIAGNOSIS: Body image disturbance related to alopecia

OUTCOME: Pt will verbalize methods of managing hair loss.

NURSING INTERVENTIONS:

1. Assess pt/SO understanding of hair loss induced by antineoplastic regimen.

2. Teach pt why hair loss occurs and what body hair will be affected (scalp, body, face).

3. Teach pt to wear hat or cap to retain body heat and cover head.

4. Pt should consider preparing for hair loss by having hair cut short before loss or thinning or purchase a wig or head coverings before hair loss.

5. Encourage pt/SO to verbalize effect of hair loss on body image.

6. If hair thinning is expected as opposed to total hair loss, teach pt to use a gentle shampoo and avoid tugging or pulling hair.

NURSING DIAGNOSIS: Fatigue related to chemotherapy

OUTCOME: Pt will use methods to promote adaptation to fatigue.

NURSING INTERVENTIONS:

1. Assess pt/SO understanding of cause of fatigue and methods of fatigue management.

2. Encourage pt/SO to verbalize impact of fatigue on usual lifestyle.

3. Encourage periods of rest and activity, midday naps, and routine times of arising and retiring, mild exercise routine, such as walking.

4. Remind pt to ask for assistance when required. Assess need for help at home (e.g., home health aide, homemaker).

5. Monitor H/H results and report low counts to physician. Treat as per hospital or clinic standard.

6. Teach pt to report incidence and severity of fatigue.

7. Teach pt to administer prescribed erythropoietin injections.

NURSING DIAGNOSIS: Risk of infection or bleeding from myelosuppression or steroids

OUTCOME: Pt will promptly notify nurse-physician of s-s of bleeding or infection. Pt will verbalize understanding of serious, potentially life-threatening nature of infection and that hospitalization may be required for IV antibiotics.

TABLE 13–5 Standard of Care: Chemotherapy for the Management of Hormone-Refractory Prostate Cancer, continued

NURSING INTERVENTIONS:

1. Assess pt/SO understanding of s-s of bleeding or infection.
2. Educate pt to notify nurse-physician of bleeding, fever, sore throat, cough, episodes of chills or diaphoresis, dysuria. Emphasize need to notify the physician promptly of s-s of infection.
3. Have pt monitor temperature each afternoon and whenever he feels warm or has the chills. Have pt keep a record of temperatures.
4. Have pt avoid infection sources such as children and adults who are sick, large crowds, pet stool, plants and flowers.
5. Pt should avoid aspirin, NSAIDs, other over-the-counter meds that contain aspirin or NSAIDs.
6. Pt should shave with electric razor and avoid other activities that may cause bleeding.
7. Obtain cultures (blood, urine, central lines), chest radiograph as ordered.
8. Administer IV antibiotics as prescribed.
9. Administer platelets as prescribed.
10. Monitor CBC differential. Calculate ANC. Notify physician when ANC < 1.0.
11. Educate pt on correct method of taking antibiotics at home.
12. Monitor pt for change in vital signs, increased temperature, RR and HR, decreasing blood pressure. Report changes to physician.
13. Arrange for home care for infusion therapy of antibiotics when pt ready for discharge.
14. Administer acetaminophen to manage fever.
15. Avoid rectal suppositories, enemas, IM injections, other procedures that violate the integrity of skin or mucous membranes.
16. Institute platelet-bleeding or neutropenic precautions when appropriate.
17. Promote good hygiene with daily bath.
18. Promote good hand-washing technique by all health care providers.
19. No fresh fruits or vegetables in diet; cooked foods should be consumed.
20. Monitor skin and mucous membranes for infection, bleeding.
21. Send stool for Hematest as ordered. Monitor urine for blood.
22. Apply pressure to venipuncture sites until bleeding stops.
23. Monitor neurologic signs for change in mental status.
24. No straining on bowel movement. Administer laxatives and stool softeners to maintain regular soft formed stools.

NURSING DIAGNOSIS: Altered comfort related to edema

OUTCOME: Pt will manage leg edema at home.

NURSING INTERVENTIONS:

1. Assess weight and edema before each treatment.
2. Educate pt to elevate legs while sitting and avoid prolonged standing.
3. Diuretics may be useful in managing leg edema.
4. Ascertain that appropriate premedications have been taken.
5. Compression stockings may be useful.

continues

TABLE 13–5 Standard of Care: Chemotherapy for the Management of Hormone-Refractory Prostate Cancer, continued

6. Educate pt to notify physician at onset of leg edema because cause may be related to DVT.

7. Drug dose may need to be modified.

NURSING DIAGNOSIS: Risk for altered nutrition related to nausea, vomiting, diarrhea. Risk for altered fluid and electrolyte balance related to vomiting, diarrhea

OUTCOME: Pt will verbalize understanding of how to manage nausea, vomiting, or diarrhea. Pt will recognize s-s of dehydration and notify physician.

NURSING INTERVENTIONS:

1. Assess pt understanding of methods to manage nausea, vomiting, and diarrhea.

2. Administer antiemetic before treatment and have pt take antiemetics on a routine basis if oral antineoplastics cause nausea at home.

3. Have pt notify physician if s-s of dehydration develop: dry mouth, reduced urine output, concentrated urine, weakness; or causes of dehydration: vomiting, diarrhea.

4. Have foods prepared in room different from where foods are consumed because odors may cause nausea.

5. Educate pt as to low-residue diet and to consume large amounts of fluids and electrolytes and use of antidiarrheal drugs if diarrhea occurs.

6. Administer antidiarrheal medication as prescribed.

7. Administer IV fluids and electrolytes as prescribed.

8. Monitor BUN and creatinine values.

9. Measure I&O; include volume of liquid stool in output.

10. Weigh twice each week.

11. Consult dietitian.

12. Keep emesis basin and commode clean and odor free.

13. Encourage resting in a quiet place.

14. Use distraction such as deep breathing, music therapy, guided imagery.

15. Keep pt NPO during vomiting episodes and slowly restart clear liquids when vomiting stops. Have pt try tea, crackers, toast, bland foods.

16. Avoid foods containing lactose, fat, and sweet or spicy foods.

17. Perform frequent mouth care and frequent perianal care after diarrhea.

NURSING DIAGNOSIS: Altered oral mucous membrane integrity

OUTCOME: Pt will be able to perform good oral care to keep mucous membranes clean and moist.

NURSING INTERVENTIONS:

1. Teach pt about good oral care: Brush teeth after meals with soft toothbrush and fluoride toothpaste and floss if it does not cause pain or bleeding. Pt should rinse mouth well with warm tap water or saline, and rinse mouth several times each day to keep mouth moist and clean.

2. Pt should consume bland low-acid diet high in protein and calories.

3. Topical analgesics or anesthetics are useful for mouth sores such as a mixture of viscous lidocaine (xylocaine), antacid, and liquid pediatric diphenhydramine mixed in a 1:1:1 solution. Use 5 ml as needed by mouth. Instruct pt to swish and spit out solution.

TABLE 13–5 Standard of Care: Chemotherapy for the Management of Hormone-Refractory Prostate Cancer, continued

    4. Encourage large fluid intake (> 2 L/day).

    5. Monitor oral cavity for pain, difficulty swallowing, sore throat, white patches, and other signs of oral infection, and notify physician. Obtain cultures as ordered.

NURSING DIAGNOSIS: Risk for altered neurologic function related to peripheral neuropathy

OUTCOME: Pt will use safety measures to reduce risk of injury.

NURSING INTERVENTIONS:

    1. Assess pt for altered sensation, altered gait.

    2. Educate pt as to safety issues, concerns related to neuropathies.

    3. Have pt wear shoes at all times to avoid foot injury.

    4. Pt should use care with sharp and hot items because sensation is reduced.

    5. Altered sensation will slowly improve over time.

    6. Pt should notify nurse of altered sensation.

    7. Pt may need assistance with tasks requiring fine motor function such as buttoning shirts.

    8. Drug doses may need to be modified because of neuropathies.

    9. Assess level of pain resulting from neuropathies and consider use of medications to reduce pain.

    10. Monitor pt for injuries.

    11. Consult PT/OT, home care as needed.

NURSING DIAGNOSIS: Risk for altered nutrition related to anorexia, taste changes

OUTCOME: Pt will verbalize understanding of how to alter foods to enhance food intake.

NURSING INTERVENTIONS:

    1. Consult with dietitian. Perform calorie counts for 3 days to assess caloric intake.

    2. Encourage pt to experiment with different flavorings, herbs, spices to promote food intake.

    3. Encourage pt to eat favorite foods.

    4. Provide high-calorie nutrient-concentrated foods that are easy to prepare and consume.

    5. Consider use of appetite-stimulating medication.

    6. Provide recipes and written information on methods of increasing calorie intake without needing to eat more food.

    7. Assess ability to obtain and prepare foods.

    8. Weigh weekly.

    9. Encourage mild exercise such as walking after consulting with physician.

    10. Encourage use of liquid diet supplements.

    11. Experiment with different foods, different culturally appropriate foods; cold, cool, or room temperature foods; and those without odor. Have family provide foods from home.

NURSING DIAGNOSIS: Risk for altered tissue perfusion

OUTCOME: Pt will have prompt recognition of s-s of anemia.

NURSING INTERVENTIONS:

    1. Educate pt as to s-s of anemia (↑HR, ↑RR, ↑fatigue, pallor, dizziness, palpitations) and need to notify nurse should these develop.

continues

TABLE 13–5 Standard of Care: Chemotherapy for the Management of Hormone-Refractory Prostate Cancer, continued

2. Monitor H/H, and report $>$ 1 g reduction in Hgb or Hgb $<$ 8.0.

3. Transfuse blood products as ordered.

4. Teach pt to change positions slowly to avoid dizziness.

5. Monitor pulse oximetry.

6. Educate pt to self-administer erythropoietin.

7. Teach pt about foods high in iron.

8. Assess need for supplemental oxygen.

NURSING DIAGNOSIS: Potential for constipation as a result of reduced mobility, decreased dietary fiber intake

OUTCOME: Pt will have an easily formed bowel movement at least every other day.

NURSING INTERVENTIONS:

1. Educate pt about need to have soft but formed, easy-to-pass stools.

2. Teach pt to take stool softeners and laxatives daily.

3. Teach pt how to titrate laxatives and stool softeners to manage bowels (increase dose with hard stools, decrease dose with diarrhea).

4. Increase amount of fiber and fluid in diet if tolerated.

5. Encourage mild exercise, such as walking, after discussion with physician.

NURSING DIAGNOSIS: Risk for cardiac toxicity

OUTCOME: Pt will promptly recognize s-s of cardiac toxicity.

NURSING INTERVENTIONS:

1. Assess pt for s-s of preexisting heart disease: chest pain, poor exercise tolerance, edema, shortness of breath, abnormal ECG, low ejection fraction, cough, JVD, ↑ or ↓ HR, extra heart sounds.

2. Monitor cumulative dose of cardiotoxic agents.

3. Educate pt to notify nurse or physician if any of these symptoms develop.

NURSING DIAGNOSIS: Risk for arthralgia, myalgia related to chemotherapy

OUTCOME: Pt will verbalize an understanding of how to manage arthralgia, myalgia.

NURSING INTERVENTIONS:

1. Educate pt as to cause of myalgia and arthralgia and its time-limited course.

2. Acetaminophen, two regular-strength tablets q 4 h PRN, may be useful in managing discomfort. Pt needs to follow package directions.

3. Pt should notify nurse if analgesic not effective.

NURSING DIAGNOSIS: Risk for *anaphylactoid* reaction related to taxane chemotherapy

OUTCOME: Pt will not experience a hypersensitivity reaction.

NURSING INTERVENTIONS:

1. Monitor vital signs before, q 15 min during, and at end of infusion.

2. Administer prescribed steroids, antihistamine, and histamine-2 blocker before infusion. *Ensure that patient has taken oral steroids as prescribed and understands need to continue steroids for the entire time prescribed.*

3. Monitor for hypotension, bronchospasm, facial flushing, dyspnea, abdominal and leg pain. Most reactions occur in the first 10 min of the infusion.

TABLE 13–5 Standard of Care: Chemotherapy for the Management of Hormone-Refractory Prostate Cancer, continued

4. Immediately terminate infusion with development of s-s of reaction and notify physician.

5. Maintain patent IV site with NSS.

6. Have emergency drugs available.

NURSING DIAGNOSIS: Risk of hemorrhagic cystitis related to cyclophosphamide therapy

OUTCOME: Pt will not experience hemorrhagic cystitis.

NURSING INTERVENTIONS:

1. Educate pt as to need to take oral drug in morning.

2. Pt needs to consume 2–3 L of fluid each day.

3. Pt needs to void hs to avoid having drug lay in bladder during night. Pt should void promptly at initial urge to void.

4. Pt needs to notify nurse or physician of hematuria promptly.

NURSING DIAGNOSIS: Risk of hepatotoxicity related to chemotherapy.

OUTCOME: Pt will have prompt recognition of s-s of hepatotoxicity.

NURSING INTERVENTIONS:

1. Assess pt for abnormal LFTs before initiation of therapy. Assess pt for history of alcohol abuse, which may promote liver toxicity.

2. Educate pt as to s-s of liver toxicity: dark urine, light-colored stool, yellow skin or sclera, itching.

3. Monitor LFT results and notify physician of abnormal results.

4. Have pt notify nurse or physician promptly if s-s of hepatotoxicity develop.

5. Drug doses may be modified in presence of altered LFT results.

6. Pt is to avoid alcohol and other drugs that may increase risk of hepatotoxicity.

NURSING DIAGNOSIS: Risk for hyperglycemia from steroid therapy

OUTCOME: The pt will have prompt recognition of s-s of hyperglycemia.

NURSING INTERVENTIONS:

1. Educate pt as to s-s of hyperglycemia: thirst, hunger, increased urination.

2. Monitor blood glucose results.

3. Notify physician of increased glucose levels.

4. Consult with dietitian regarding diabetic diet.

5. Institute diabetic education.

6. Set up home visits by visiting nurse.

NURSING DIAGNOSIS: Potential for injury due to ocular toxicities

OUTCOME: Patient will have prompt recognition and treatment of excess tearing and other ocular toxicities.

NURSING INTERVENTIONS:

1. Assess for tearing and history of eye disorders at baseline and prior to each treatment.

2. Refer patient for ophthalmology evaluation if history of eye problems present, at baseline and routinely for patients receiving weekly docetaxel and as needed for patients receiving docetaxel every 2 or 3 weeks.

3. Artificial tears should be used.

continues

TABLE 13–5 Standard of Care: Chemotherapy for the Management of Hormone-Refractory Prostate Cancer, continued

4. Risk of ocular toxicities increases the longer the patient receives therapy with docetaxel.

NURSING DIAGNOSIS: Potential for injury due to thromboembolic events

OUTCOME: Patient will not experience a thromboembolic event.

NURSING INTERVENTIONS:

1. Educate patient as to need to take prescribed aspirin, warfarin, or both.
2. Educate patient to report symptoms of DVT, PE, or other thrombotic or embolic events immediately and to call for emergency treatment.
3. Educate patient to monitor for bleeding.

PT, patient; SO, significant other; LFTs, liver function tests; H/H, hematocrit and hemoglobin; IV, intravenous; NSAIDs, nonsteroidal anti-inflammatory drugs; meds, medications; CBC, complete blood cell count; ANC, absolute neutrophil count; IM, intramuscular; DVT, deep vein thrombosis; BUN, blood urea nitrogen; I & O, intake and output; NPO, nothing by mouth; RR, respiration rate; HR, heart rate; Hgb, hemoglobin; ECG, electrocardiogram; JVD, jugular venous distention; T, temperature; hs, at bedtime; s-s, signs-symptoms; NSS, normal saline solution. Carpenito-Moyet,[33] Barton-Burke,[34] Wilkes,[35] Schulmeister,[36] Tortorice,[37] Higano et al.,[38] Esmaeli et al.,[39] Sinibaldi, et al.,[31] Lubiniecki et al.[84]

Source: Held-Warmkessel, J. Treatment of hormone-refractory prostate cancer with chemotherapy. In: Held-Warmkessel, J., ed. *Contemporary Issues in Prostate Cancer: A Nursing Perspective* (2nd ed). Jones and Bartlett Publishers, 2006, 284–317. Reprinted with permission by Jones and Bartlett Publishers.

References

1. Smaletz O, Scher HI, Small EJ, et al. Nomogram for overall survival of patients with progressive metastatic prostate cancer after castration. *J Clin Oncol.* 2002;20: 3972–3982.
2. Small EJ, Halabi S, Dawson NA, et al. Antiandrogen withdrawal alone or in combination with ketoconazole in androgen-independent prostate cancer patients: a phase III trial (CALGB9583). *J Clin Oncol.* 2004;22:1025–1033.
3. Petrylak DP, Tangen CM, Hussain MHA, et al. Docetaxel and estramustine compared with mitoxantrone and prednisone for advanced refractory prostate cancer. *N Engl J Med.* 2004;351:1513–1520.
4. Tannock IF, de Wit R, Berry WR, et al. Docetaxel plus prednisone or mitoxantrone plus prednisone for advanced prostate cancer. *N Engl J Med.* 2004;351:1502–1512.
5. Moore MJ, Tannock IF. Overview of Canadian trials in hormonally resistant prostate cancer. *Semin Oncol.* 1996;23(6, suppl 14):15–19.
6. Esper PS, Pienta KJ. Supportive care in the patient with hormone refractory prostate cancer. *Semin Urol Oncol.* 1997;15:56–64.
7. Scher HI, Steineck G, Kelly WK. Hormone-refractory (D3) prostate cancer: refining the concept. *Urology.* 1995;46:142–148.
8. Bubley GJ, Carducci M, Dahut W, et al. Eligibility and response guidelines for phase II clinical trials in androgen-independent prostate cancer: recommendations from the Prostate-Specific Antigen Working Group. *J Clin Oncol.* 1999;17:3461–3467.
9. Martel CL, Gumerlock PH, Meyers FJ, et al. Current strategies in the management of hormone refractory prostate cancer. *Cancer Treat Rev.* 2003;29:171–187.

10. Raghavan D, Coorey G, Rosen M, et al. Management of hormone-resistant prostate cancer: an Australian trial. *Semin Oncol.* 1996;23(6, suppl 14):20–23.
11. Iversen P, Rasmussen F, Asmussen C, et al. Estramustine phosphate versus placebo as a second line treatment after orchiectomy in patients with metastatic prostate cancer: DAPROCA study 9002. *J Urol.* 1997;157:929–934
12. Roth BJ, Yeap BY, Wilding G, et al. Taxol in hormone-refractory carcinoma of the prostate. *Cancer* 1993;72:2457–2460.
13. Hussain MH, Pienta KJ, Redman BG, et al. Oral etoposide in the treatment of hormone-refractory prostate cancer. *Cancer.* 1994;74:100–103.
14. Kojima T, Shimazui T, Onozawa M, et al. Weekly administration of docetaxel in patients with hormone-refractory prostate cancer: a pilot study on Japanese patients. *Jpn J Clin Oncol.* 2004;34:137–141.
15. Schultz M, Wei J, Picus J. A phase II trial of docetaxel in patients with hormone refractory prostate cancer (HRPC) [abstract 1320]. *Proc Am Soc Clin Oncol.* 1998;17:342a.
16. Trivedi C, Redman B, Flaherty LE, et al. Weekly 1-hour infusion of paclitaxel: clinical feasibility and efficacy in patients with hormone-refractory prostate carcinoma. *Cancer.* 2000;89:431–436.
17. Raghavan D, Cox K, Pearson BS, et al. Oral cyclophosphamide for the management of hormone-refractory prostate cancer. *Br J Urol.* 1993;72:625–628.
18. Moore MJ, Osoba D, Murphy K, et al. Use of palliative endpoints to evaluate the effects of mitoxantrone and low-dose prednisone in patients with hormonally resistant prostate cancer. *J Clin Oncol.* 1994;12:689–694.
19. Tannock IF, Osoba D, Stockler MR, et al. Chemotherapy with mitoxantrone plus prednisone or prednisone alone for symptomatic hormone-resistant prostate cancer: a Canadian randomized trial with palliative end points. *J Clin Oncol.* 1996;14:1756–1764.
20. Kantoff PW, Halabi S, Conaway M, et al. Hydrocortisone with or without mitoxantrone in men with hormone refractory prostate cancer : results of the Cancer and Leukemia Group B study 9182 study. *J Clin Oncol.* 1999;17:2506–2525.
21. Sheen W-C, Chen J-S, Wang H-M, et al. A modified low-dose regimen of mitoxantrone and prednisolone in patients with androgen-independent prostate cancer. *Jpn J Clin Oncol.* 2004;34:337–341.
22. Ernst DS, Tannock IF, Winguist EW, et al. Randomized, double-blind, controlled trial of mitoxantrone/prednisone and clondronate versus mitoxantrone/prednisone and placebo in patients with hormone-refractory prostate cancer and pain. *J Clin Oncol.* 2003;21:3335–3342.
23. Berry W, Dakhil S, Modiano M, et al. Phase III study of mitoxantrone plus low dose prednisone versus low dose prednisone alone in patients with asymptomatic hormone refractory prostate cancer. *J Urol.* 2002;168:2439–2443.
24. DeConti R, Balducci L, Einstein A, et al. A phase II trial of mitoxantrone/paclitaxel in hormone-refractory prostate cancer [abstract 1270]. *Pr Am Soc Clin Oncol.* 1998;17:329a.
25. Pienta KJ, Redman BG, Bandekar R, et al. A phase II trial of oral estramustine and oral etoposide in hormone refractory prostate cancer. *Urology.* 1997;50:401–407.
26. Kreis W, Budman DR, Fetten J, et al. Phase I trial of the combination of daily estramustine phosphate and intermittent docetaxel in patients with metastatic hormone refractory prostate cancer. *Ann Oncol.* 1999;10:33–38.
27. Kreis W, Budman D. Daily oral estramustine and intermittent intravenous docetaxel (Taxotere) as chemotherapeutic treatment for metastatic, hormone-refractory prostate cancer. *Sem Oncol.* 1999;26(suppl 17):34–38.

28. Petrylak DP, Macarthur R, O'Connor J, et al. Phase I/II studies of docetaxel (taxotere) combined with estramustine in men with hormone-refractory prostate cancer. *Sem Oncol.* 1999;26(suppl 17):28–33.
29. Savarese, DM, Halabi S, Hars V, et al. Phase II study of docetaxel, estramustine, and low-dose hydrocortisone in men with hormone-refractory prostate cancer: a final report of CALGB 9780. *J Clin Oncol.* 2001;19: 2509–2516.
30. Sitka Copur M, Ledakis P, Lynch J, et al. Weekly docetaxel and estramustine in patients with hormone-refractory prostate cancer. *Sem Oncol.* 2001; 28: 16–21.
31. Sinibaldi VJ, Carducci MA, Moore-Cooper S, et al. Phase II evaluation of docetaxel plus one-day oral estramustine phosphate in the treatment of patients with androgen independent prostate cancer. *Cancer.* 2002;94:1457–1465.
32. Eymard J-C, Joly F, Priou F, et al. Phase II randomized trial of docetaxel plus estramustine (DE) versus docetaxel (D) in patients (pts) with hormone-refractory prostate cancer (HRPC): a final report [abstract 4603]. *Proc Am Soc Clin Oncol.* 2004;23:406.
33. Carpentio-Moyet LJ. *Nursing Diagnosis: Application to Clinical Practice.* 10th ed. Philadelphia, Pa: Lippincott; 2004.
34. Barton-Burke MB, Wilkes GM, Ingwersen KC, et al. *Cancer Chemotherapy: A Nursing Process Approach.* 3rd ed. Sudbury, Mass: Jones and Bartlett; 2001.
35. Wilkes GM. Potential toxicities and nursing management. In: Barton-Burke MB, Wilkes GM, Ingwersen KC, eds. *Cancer Chemotherapy: A Nursing Process Approach.* 3rd ed. Sudbury, Mass: Jones and Bartlett; 2001:89–186.
36. Schulmeister L. Nutrition. In: Otto SE, ed. *Oncology Nursing.* 4th ed. St. Louis, MO: CV Mosby; 2001:843–864.
37. Tortorice PV. *Chemotherapy: Principles of Therapy.* In: Yarbro CH, Frogge MH, Goodman M, et al., eds. *Cancer Nursing: Principles and Practice.* 5th ed. Sudbury, Mass: Jones and Bartlett; 2000:352–384.
38. Higano CS, Beer TM, Garzotto M, et al. Need for awareness and monitoring of ocular toxicities (OT) due to weekly docetaxel administration: experience during a trial of neoadjuvant docetaxel (D) and mitoxantrone (M) for patients with high-risk prostate cancer (PC)[abstract 4577]. *J Clin Oncol.* 2004;22:401–405.
39. Esmaeli B, Hidaji L, Adinin RB, et al. Blockage of the lacrimal drainage apparatus as a side effect of docetaxel therapy. *Cancer.* 2003;98:504–507.
40. Lubiniecki GM, Berlin JA, Weinstein RB, et al. Thromboembolic events with estramustine phosphate-based chemotherapy in patients with hormone-refractory prostate carcinoma: results of a meta-analysis. *Cancer.* 2004;101:2755–2759.

Part IV

Quality of Life Issues

Chapter 14

Quality of Life and Prostate Cancer

PHYSICAL WELL-BEING[1-5]

- Treatment selected will impact patient's remaining life span and affect his quality of life during that time
- Radical prostatectomy patients are affected by incontinence and impotence more frequently than men who receive radiation therapy.
- Changes in bowel function are more common in men who receive radiation therapy.
- There may not be any difference in the health-related quality of life (QOL) between men who undergo surgery or radiation.

URINARY MORBIDITY[6-32]

Symptoms

- Dysuria (most common)
- Hematuria (transient, managed with increased fluid intake)
- Frequency
- Urgency
- Hesitancy
- Urinary retention
- Incontinence

Severity

- Mild to moderate in majority
- 11–22% experience severe symptoms

Dysuria

- Varies in severity from irritation to burning
- Urine specimen should be sent to rule out a urinary tract infection.
- Ibuprofen is often effective
- Phenazopyridine may also be used
- Patient should increase fluid intake, and avoid urinary tract irritants such as caffeine and alcohol

Urinary Incontinence

- Incidence after prostatectomy—up to 94% of patients become continent 18 months after surgery, but 2–87% continue to have problems with incontinence
- Incidence after radiation therapy is lower
- Rates vary based on definition of incontinence used in the research study
- Rates higher after prostatectomy than after radiation therapy, but rates of distress due to incontinence are similar

Problems associated with incontinence
- Urine leakage
- Leakage with sneezing, coughing
- Problems with sexuality
- Need to use incontinence devices
- Psychosocial distress—anxiety, hopelessness, loss of control, embarrassment, low self-esteem, depression, anger, shame, sensitivity, social isolation, avoidance of intimacy

Types of incontinence

Stress incontinence
- Results from increase in intra-abdominal pressure
- Related to distal urethral sphincter incompetence with increased pressure such as sneezing and coughing
- Most common cause of postprostatectomy incontinence

Urge incontinence
- Urgency, related to detrusor instability, bladder inability to store urine, bladder spasms, low bladder compliance, sensory urgency, and fistula
- Less common single cause of incontinence after prostatectomy
- Symptoms include urgency and frequency
- May occur along with bladder dysfunction, sphincter incompetence, and stress incontinence

Overflow incontinence
- Inability to empty bladder completely, resulting in incontinence
- Associated with frequency and feeling of incomplete bladder emptying
- Uncommon cause of incontinence after prostatectomy

Functional incontinence
- Due to physical or mental disability interfering with ability to reach or use toilet
- Uncommon cause of incontinence after prostatectomy

Incontinence Assessment

- Goal—Determine symptoms, frequency of incontinent episodes, continent episodes, fluid intake, amount of urine voided with continent and incontinent episodes, use of incontinence devices and outcome, precipitating factors
- Have patient keep a diary of information. This information is useful in determining the cause of incontinence and developing an incontinence plan for patient treatment

Baseline data useful in determining effect of interventions
- Physical assessment—Tone of abdominal and rectal muscles provides information needed for pelvic muscle exercises
- Diagnostic studies—Postvoid residuals and cystogram are used to assess bladder function and contractions and incontinence

Initial interventions
- Consume 48–64 ounces of liquid per day; no alcohol, caffeine, or other bladder irritants
- Stress and urge incontinence are often both involved in postprostatectomy incontinence
- Often responds to behavioral interventions and education

Nursing Interventions

- Assessment of patient's goal for incontinence management, knowledge of incontinence, social support, and manual dexterity
- Patient education must be done frequently including both formal and informal approaches and need to include partner

Pelvic muscle exercises (PMEs) or Kegel exercises
- Goal is to strengthen pubococcygeal muscles resulting in improved urethral resistance and reduced incontinence
- Stress incontinence and possibly urge incontinence improve
- Crucial that patient contracts correct muscle during exercise
- Patient education is accomplished verbally and by use of biofeedback
- Begun about 4 weeks after surgery; patients using biofeedback progress at their own pace to learn muscle exercises
- Biofeedback uses monitor and external electrodes to communicate information about pubococcygeal muscle activity
- Both office treatments and home treatments may be used
- Effective in about 95% of patients

Bladder training and voiding schedules
- Schedule timed voiding in a progressive manner lengthening time between voidings to the goal of voiding every 3–4 hours
- Includes monitoring and recording fluid intake, distraction, and relaxation techniques

Pelvic floor electrical stimulation
- To improve urethral resistance, reduce bladder contractility, and strengthen weak pelvic muscles

Pharmacologic interventions
- See **Table 14–1** for drugs used in incontinence management
- When used in the elderly, risk of side effects is greater, especially confusion, tachycardia, urinary retention, postural hypotension, hallucinations and nightmares
- Assess patient for side effects and educate patient as to self-care measures to manage dry mouth, constipation, and other side effects
- Assess patient for visual disturbances and educate patient about safety measures

Artificial sphincters
- Used when other interventions unsuccessful and incontinence is debilitating
- Bladder pressure must be under control prior to surgery
- Device surgically placed in bladder neck
- Side effects—infection, incontinence, device erosion

Condom catheter or external collecting pouch
- Device is placed on outside of penis to collect urine
- Applied to clean, dry skin avoiding areas of pressure
- Replaced every 1–2 days
- Assess skin daily for dermatitis, maceration, ischemia, and obstruction
- Side effects—irritation, penile constriction

Penile clamps
- Externally compress urethra
- Must be released every 2 hours for voiding and to reduce pressure on urethra, and immediately for any pain or discomfort. May be uncomfortable

TABLE 14-1 Pharmacologic Therapy for Stress-Urge Incontinence

Drug	Dose	Indications	Side Effects
Anticholinergics and antimuscarinics*			
Oxybutynin	2.5–5 mg tid-qid	Direct relaxant effect on detrusor muscle. AHRQ recommended anticholinergic drug of choice for treatment of detrusor instability	Dry mouth*, + blurred vision, + constipation+
Oxytrol (transdermal)	3.9 mg/day	Same as oxybutynin	Same as oxybutynin
Propantheline (synthetic analogue of atropine with pure anticholinergic properties)	7.5–30 mg 3–5 times/day up to 60 mg qid	Recommended second-line agent for urge incontinence secondary to detrusor instability in men who can tolerate full dosage	Headache, xerostomia+ blurred vision+ drowsiness, constipation, tachycardia, inhibition of gut motility, dizziness+
Dicyclomine (synthetic antimuscarinic with direct smooth muscle relaxant)	10–20 mg bid	May be used as alternative agent to propantheline for urge incontinence	
Tolterodine tartrate	2 mg bid or 4 mg extended release	Urge incontinence	Headache, + dry mouth+
Antidepressants ±			
Tricyclic			
Imipramine	10–25 mg 1–3 times/day, increased to a maximum of 150 mg/day; less frequent administration often possible because of half-life	Urine storage facilitated by decreasing bladder contractility and increasing resistance	Dry mouth, + blurred vision, constipation
Doxepin	Used interchangeably with imipramine; 50 mg qhs with or without 25 mg in the am		Gut motility inhibition, arrhythmias, drowsiness, and confusion at higher doses; weakness, fatigue, and orthostatic hypotension may be marked in elderly; anxiety, anorexia

+ most common

*Anticholinergics are AHRQ recommended first-line therapy for patients with detrusor instability. These drugs act on muscarinic and acetylcholine receptors throughout the bladder, suppressing involuntary as well as normal contractions, which result in urge incontinence.

‡Widely used in the treatment of urge incontinence, especially nocturnal incontinence.

±These drugs act at α-adrenoceptors in the bladder neck, base, and proximal urethra, treating the urethral sphincter insufficiency that causes stress incontinence.

tid, 3 times/day, qid, 4 times/day, AHRQ, Agency for Healthcare Research and Quality; bid, 2 times/day; qhs, every bedtime.

Source: King CR. Quality of life and prostate cancer. In Held-Warmkessel J, ed. *Contemporary Issues in Prostate Cancer: A Nursing Perspective* (2nd ed). Jones and

- May not be used at night
- Pressure may cause tissue damage
- Useful during physical activity that results in incontinence

Incontinence pads and undergarments
- May encourage dependence and prevent patient from seeking treatment for incontinence
- Disposable and reusable devices available
- Useful in postoperative period and when physical activity produces incontinence
- Expensive when used for long periods of time
- Skin at risk of altered integrity from exposure to urine
- Good skin care required with barrier skin protectants

BOWEL DYSFUNCTION[33–45]

Introduction
- More common in men treated with radiation therapy
- Impact on QOL minor
- Symptoms include diarrhea, urgency, crampy abdominal pain, and bleeding with bowel movements

Acute Side Effects
- Diarrhea, rectal urgency, pain with bowel movement
- Develops in 60% of patients during third week of treatment and needs some form of drug management
- Managed with antidiarrheals (see Chapter 10) and patient education

Chronic Side Effects
- Radiation proctitis with diarrhea, fecal incontinence, rectal pain, tenesmus, rectal bleeding, anal stricture, and fistula
- Incidence: 5–19%

Chronic Radiation Proctopathy
- Alteration in rectal mucosa, connective tissue fibrosis and/or arteriole endarteritis and is accompanied by symptoms and develops 3 months after completion of radiation therapy
- Diagnosed by endoscopic examination of bowel
- More serious is bleeding that develops 6 months to 2 years after completion of radiation therapy
- Caused by friable mucosal angiectasis
- Bleeding occurs spontaneously or with bowel movements; clots may be present; may occur daily or intermittently
- Treatment—topically administered steroid enemas, sucralfate enemas, or formalin enemas
- Laser coagulation of angioectatic lesions
- Surgery—treatment of last resort or for obstruction, perforation, or fistula
- Bowel resection or colostomy
- Hyperbaric oxygen treatment

PSYCHOLOGICAL WELL-BEING
- As equally an important factor in QOL as physical well-being

SOCIAL WELL-BEING

- Requires frequent nursing assessment throughout diagnosis, treatment, and posttreatment
- Nurses need to assess support systems, financial needs, coping, and sexual functioning
- Patients should be referred as needed to assist them with adapting

SEXUAL DYSFUNCTION[1, 4, 13, 33, 35, 36, 46–69]

Introduction

- Defined as a wide range of alterations in sexuality from loss of libido to inability to attain or maintain an erection satisfactory for intercourse
- Includes changes in orgasm, nocturnal erections, and desire for sexual activity
- Functioning may be reduced by aging, but its importance may not change
- Dysfunction may cause depression, anxiety, poor self-image, poor self-esteem, and affect the relationship with partner
- Alterations in sexuality affect men who have received radiation therapy, hormonal therapy, and prostatectomy
- These alterations are unlikely to change patient treatment decisions when asked if same treatment would be repeated
- Patients may not include altered sexuality in their view of the impact of treatment on their quality of life
- Prostatectomy patients have more sexual dysfunction than men who have received treatment with radiation therapy
- Larger fields of radiation have a greater impact on erectile dysfunction than three-dimensional conformal therapy
- Impotency rates for men after prostatectomy are as high as 85% at 3 months and 75% at 12 months compared with 11% prior to surgery. Some improvement in erectile function may be seen with time
- Impotency rates after radiation therapy are lower than after surgery and do have an impact on the patient's QOL. Changes are noted approximately 12 months after radiation therapy
- Changes noted by patients include alterations in desire, erectile capability.
- Risk factors for erectile dysfunction (ED) after radiation therapy—older age, size of treatment field, dose and fractionation schedule
- Risk factors for ED after surgery—age, preoperative ED, tumor size, type of procedure, altered penile blood supply, tumor growth into seminal vesicles, atherosclerosis
- Include patient and partner in all education regarding alterations in sexuality resulting from treatment
- Refer for counseling as appropriate

Assessment for Sexual Dysfunction

- Critical to determine impact of erectile dysfunction on patients QOL and relationships
- Should be performed on a routine basis during routine patient assessments

Management of Erectile Dysfunction

- Multidisciplinary approach to management of ED—need to consider medical and psychosocial aspects
- Try least invasive methods first
- There needs to be good communication between the patient and his partner

Vacuum constriction devices
- A plastic cylinder is placed around penis; scrotal skin is carefully pulled away
- Suction is applied to pull blood into penis
- Constriction band is applied to base of penis to contain blood for 30 minutes
- Motivation, manual dexterity, and practice sessions are required prior to use
- Effective in about 89% of users

Side effects
- Related to constriction band, length of time band is applied to penis—reduced skin temperature, numbness, cyanosis, increased girth, blocked ejaculation, pain
- Related to pumping too quickly—pain and pulling on scrotal tissues
- Related to pumping to too high a pressure—petechiae and ecchymoses

Patient education
- Practice required prior to use—applying band correctly so it is not too loose or too tight, using device, pump to 100 mm Hg, being careful not to pump too quickly or to high pressures. Practice with pumping prior to practicing applying band; practice with amount of constriction band tightness needed to maintain erection; easier to apply to partially erect penis
- Avoid use of aspirin, other salicylates, and nonsteroidal anti-inflammatory drugs; caution with anticoagulants and thrombocytopenia
- Generous use of lubricants after band applied and not before
- Follow-up required for answering questions and providing support and encouragement
- Support group participation may be helpful
- Partner support is an important component
- Device failure with a given patient is due to pain, discomfort, and premature loss of erection

Intracavernosal injections
- Effective in 90% of patients
- Drug injected into corpora cavernosa to produce erection
- Agents used have vasoactive effect—prostaglandin E, papaverine, and phentolamine
- May be used alone or in combination; dose and volume of each drug are lower when used in combination and when used with sexual stimulation
- Injection side effects
  - Minor—pain; ecchymosis; infection (rare); prolonged erections in 10% of patients during dose titration period; increased liver function tests
  - Major—fibrotic changes, nodule or plaque formation in tissue in 31%; incidence is lower with prostaglandin E; vasovagal reactions, hypotension, or hypertension during dose titration period
- Injection candidates—patient finds this type of therapy acceptable; good manual dexterity; vision acceptable; not obese; no cardiovascular or cerebrovascular disease; no priapism or penile fibrosis, increased liver function tests, or sickle cell trait or disease
- Patient education
  - Length of time commitment—for dose titration, waiting for loss of erection in clinic
  - Side effects—major and minor
  - Need for erection reversal if erection lasts longer than 3–4 hours

Transurethral prostaglandin E
- Drug placed in urethra; produces erection lasting up to 1 hour
- Effective in 70% of patients after prostatectomy
- Dose: 125–250 mcg, titrated up to 500–1000 mcg
- Side effects—pain, burning, hematuria, dizziness, hypotension, and priapism
- Patient education
  - Hold penis upright
  - Insert drug using applicator, and insert 3 cm into urethra
  - To improve drug absorption—rub penis for ½ minute
  - To reduce pain or stinging—rub penis until discomfort resolves

Sildenafil
- Usually well tolerated
- Improves blood flow to penis
- Must be accompanied by sexual stimulation; drug does not work alone
- Dose: 25–100 mg po 1 hour prior to sexual intercourse, one dose per day maximum
- Effective in 69% of patients
- May be useful in patients who underwent bilateral nerve-sparing prostatectomy, but additional research is required
- Side effects—headache, facial flushing, dyspepsia, nasal congestion, and blue-tinged vision changes
- Absolute contraindication—oral nitrates, transdermal nitrates. Deaths have occurred with combinations
- Patient education—not to exceed dose or frequency prescribed; never to be taken with nitrates; other potential side effects. In patients with history of hypotension, may cause hypotension

Penile prosthesis
- For patients who have not responded to other interventions
- Requires surgical placement of device used to produce erections
- Different types are available—semirigid, malleable, and inflatable, also one piece or multiple pieces
- Side effects—device failure, infection, and device erosion
- Patient education—penis cannot lay flaccid due to presence of implant; after implantation—penis is shorter; other treatments for ED cannot be used; implant may need to be removed if infection develops. Reoperations may be required

SPIRITUAL WELL-BEING
- Should be assessed for its impact on the patient

QUALITY OF LIFE IN ADVANCED PROSTATE CANCER[70-71]
- Hormonal therapy affects sexual, emotional, and physical well-being.
- Side effects include loss of libido, erectile dysfunction, gynecomastia, hot flashes, and nausea (see Chapter 12).
- At advanced stages of metastatic disease, hormonal therapy may negatively affect QOL.

References
1. Talcott JA, Reiker P, Clark JA et al. Patient-reported symptoms after primary therapy for early prostate cancer. Results of a prospective cohort study. *J Clin Oncol.* 1998;16:275–283.

2. Litwin MS, Hays RO, Fink A et al. Quality-of-life outcomes in men treated for local-ized prostate cancer. *JAMA.* 1995;273:129–135.

3. Fowler F, Barry J, Lu-Yao G. Patient reported complications and follow-up treatment after radical prostatectomy. The National Medicare Experience: 1988–1990. *Urology.* 1993;42:622–629.

4. Litwin MS, Hays RO, Fink A. Quality of life outcomes in men treated for localized prostate cancer. *JAMA.* 1995;273:129–135.

5. Schapira MM, Lawrence WF, Katz DA, McAuliffe TL, Nattinger AB. Effect of treatment on quality of life among men with clinically localized prostate cancer. *Med Care.* 2001;39:243–253.

6. Fossa S, Woehre H, Kurth KH, et al. Influence of urological morbidity on quality of life in patients with prostate cancer. *Eur Urol.* 1997;31:3–8.

7. Abel L, Dafoe-Lambie J, Butler WM, Merrick GS. Treatment outcomes and quality-of-life for patients treated with prostate brachytherapy. *Clin J Oncol Nurs.* 2003; 7:48–54.

8. Chang M, Joseph A. Evolution of a bladder behavior clinic for patients after prosta-tectomy. *Urol Nurs.* 1993;13:62–66.

9. Gallo M, Fallon P, Staskin D. Urinary incontinence: Steps to evaluation, diagnosis, and treatment. *Nurse Practitioner.* 1997;22:21–41.

10. Palmer MH, Fogarty LA, Somerfield MR, Powel LL. Incontinence after prostatec-tomy: coping with incontinence after prostate cancer surgery. *Oncol Nurs Forum.* 2003;30:229–238

11. Nasr S, Ouslander J. Urinary incontinence in the elderly: causes and treatment op-tions. *Drug Aging.* 1988;12:349–360.

12. Herr HW, Kornblith AB, Ofman U. A comparison of the quality of life of patients with metastatic prostate cancer who received or did not receive hormonal therapy. *Cancer.* 1993;71:1143–1150.

13. Braslis KG, Santa-Cruz C, Brickman AI, Soloway MS. Quality of life 12 months after radical prostatectomy. *Br J Urol.* 1995;75:48–53.

14. Newman D, Burns P. Significance and impact of urinary incontinence. *Nurse Practi-tioner Forum.* 1994;5:130–133.

15. Leach GE, Trockman B, Wong A. Post-prostatectomy incontinence: Urodynamic findings and treatment outcomes. *J Urol.* 1996;155:1256–1259.

16. Bengtson J, Chapin MD, Kohli N, Loughlin KR, Seligson J, Gharib S. Urinary inconti-nence: guide to diagnosis and management. Boston (Mass): Brigham and Women's Hospital; 2004. National Guideline Clearinghouse. http://www.guideline.gov/ Accessed May 16, 2006.

17. Ficazola M, Nitti V. The etiology of post-radical prostatectomy incontinence and cor-relation of symptoms with urodynamic findings. *J Urol.* 1998;160:1317–1320.

18. Foote J, Yun S, Leach GE. Prostatectomy incontinence: pathophysiology, evaluation and management. *Urol Clin North Am.* 1991;18:229–241.

19. Harris J. Treatment of postprostatectomy urinary incontinence with behavioral meth-ods. *Clin Nurse Specialist.* 1997;11:159–166.

20. Beckman N. An overview of urinary incontinence in adults: assessments and behav-ioral interventions. *Clinical Nurse Specialist.* 1995;9:241–248.

21. Wyman J, Fantl J. Bladder training in ambulatory care management of urinary incon-tinence. *Urol Nurs.* 1991;11:11–17.

22. Agency for Health Care Policy and Research. Quick reference guide for clinicians: managing acute and chronic urinary incontinence. *J Am Acad Nurse Practitioners.* 1996;8:390–403.

23. Meaglia JP, Joseph AC, Chang M, Schmidt JD. Post-prostatectomy urinary incontinence. Response to behavioral training. *J Urol.* 1990;144:674–676.
24. Burgio KL, Strutzmn RE, Engel BT. Behavioral training for post-prostatectomy urinary incontinence. *J Urol.* 1989;141:303–306.
25. Wyman J. Comprehensive assessment and management of urinary incontinence by continence nurse specialists. *Nurse Practitioner Forum.* 1994;5:177–185.
26. Messick G, Powe C. Applying behavioral research to incontinence. *Ostomy/Wound Management.* 1997;43:40–46,48.
27. Denis P. Methodology of biofeedback. *Eur J Gastrenterol Hepatol.* 1996;8:530–533.
28. Wein A. Pharmacologic options for the overactive bladder. *Urology.* 1998;51:43–47.
29. Owens R, Karram M. Comparative tolerability of drug therapies used to treat incontinence and enuresis. *Drug Safety.* 1998;19:123–139.
30. Moore K, Richardson V. Pharmacology: impact on bladder function. *Ostomy/Wound Management.* 1998;44:30–45.
31. Kreder K, Webster G. Evaluation and management of incontinence after implantation of the artificial sphincter. *Urol Clin North Am.* 1991;18:375–381.
32. Yalla S. Management of urinary incontinence—progress and innovative strategies [editorial]. *J Urol.* 1998;159:1520–1522.
33. Shrader-Bogen CL, Kjellberg JL, McPherson CP, Murray CL. Quality of life and treatment outcomes: prostate carcinoma patients' perspectives after prostatectomy or radiation therapy. *Cancer.* 1997;79:1977–1986.
34. Yarbro CH, Ferrans CE. Quality of life of patients with prostate cancer treated with surgery or radiation therapy. *Oncol Nurs Forum.* 1998;25:685–693.
35. Beard CJ, Propert KJ, Rieker PP. Complications after treatment with external-beam irradiation in early-stage prostate cancer patients: a prospective multi-institutional outcomes study. *J Clin Oncol.* 1997;15:223–229.
36. Caffo O, Fellin G, Graffer U, Luciani L. Assessment of quality of life after radical radiotherapy for prostate cancer. *Br J Urol.* 1996;78:557–563.
37. Altwein J, Ekman P, Barry M. How is quality of life in prostate cancer patients influenced by modern treatment? The Wallengberg symopsium. *Urology.* 1997;49:66–76.
38. Soffen E, Hanks G, Hunt M, Epstein B. Conformal static field radiation therapy of early prostate cancer versus non-conformal techniques. a reduction in acute morbidity. *Int J Radiat Oncol Biol Phys.* 1992;24:485–488.
39. Cho KH, Lee CK, Levitt SH. Proctitis after conventional external radiation therapy for prostate cancer: Importance of minimizing posterior rectal dose. *Radiology.* 1995;195:699–703.
40. Lawton CA, Won MM, Pilepich MV. Long-term treatment sequelae following external beam irridation for adenocarcinoma of the prostate: Analysis of RTOG studies 7506 and 7706. Int J Radiat Oncol Biol Phys. 1991;21:935–939.
41. Swaroop VS, Gostout C. Endoscopic treatment of chronic radiation proctopathy. *J Clin Gastroenterol.* 1998;27:36–40.
42. Chapius P, Dent O, Bokey E. The development of a treatment protocol for patients with chronic radiation-induced rectal bleeding. *Aust New Zeal J Surg.* 1996;66:680–685.
43. Woo TC, Joseph D, Oxer H. Hyperbaric oxygen treatment for radiation proctitis. *Int J Radiat Oncol Biol Phys.* 1997;38:619–622.
44. Warren DC, Feehan P, Slade JB, Cianci PE. Chronic radiation proctitis treated with hyperbaric oxygen. *Undersea Hyperbaric Medicine.* 1997;24:181–184.
45. Hogan C. The nurse's role in diarrhea management. *Oncol Nurs Forum.* 1998;25:879–886.

46. Hughes MK. Sexuality issues: keeping your cool. *Oncol Nurs Forum*. 1996;23: 1597–1600.
47. Helgason A, Fredrikson M, Adolfsson J, Steinback G. Decreased sexual capacity after external radiation therapy for prostate cancer impairs quality of life. *Int J Radiat Oncol Biol Phys*. 1995;35:33–39.
48. Quallich SA, Ohl DA. Penile prostheses: patient teaching and perioperative care. Urol Nurs. 2002;22:81–92.
49. Shell JA. Evidence-based practice for symptom management in adults with cancer: Sexual dysfunction. *Oncol Nurs Forum*. 2002;29:53–69.
50. Cleary PD, Morrissey G, Oster G. Health-related quality of life in patients with advanced prostate cancer: a multinational perspective. *Qual Life Res*. 1995;4:207–220.
51. Perez MA, Meyerowitz BE, Lieskovsky G, Skinner DG, Reynolds B, Skinner EC. Quality of life and sexuality following radical prostatectomy in patients with prostate cancer who use or do not use erectile aids. *Urology*. 1997;50:740–746.
52. Zinreich ES, Derogatis LR, Herpst J. Pre- and post-treatment evaluation of sexual function in patients with adenocarcinoma of the prostate. *Int J Radiat Oncol Biol Phys*. 1990;19:729–732.
53. Borghede G, Sullivan M. Measurement of quality of life in localized prostatic cancer patients treated with radiotherapy. Development of a prostate cancer specific module supplementing the EORTC of QLQ-C30. *Qual Life Res*. 1996;5:212–222.
54. Roach M, Chinn DM, Holland J, Clarke M. A pilot survey of sexual function and quality of life following 3D conformal radiotherapy for clinically localized prostate cancer. *Int J Radiat Oncol Biol Phys*. 1996;35:869–874.
55. Hall MC. Management of erectile dysfunction after radical prostatectomy. *Sem in Urol Oncol*. 1995;13:215–223.
56. Turner LA, Althof AE, Levine SB et al. Treating erectile dysfuntion with external vacuum devices: impact upon sexual, psychological and marital functioning. *J Urol*. 1990;144:79–82.
57. Nadig P. Vacuum devices for erectile dysfunction. *Prob Urol*. 1991;5:559–565.
58. Sidi A, Becher E, Zhang G, Lewis J. Patient acceptance of and satisfaction with an external negative pressure device for impotence. *J Urol*. 1990;144:1154–1156.
59. Burnett A. Erectile dysfunction. A practical approach for primary care. *Geriatrics*. 1998;53:34–48.
60. Lewis R. The pharmacologic erection. *Prob Urol*. 1991;5:541–558.
61. Godschalk M, Chen J, Katz P, Mulligan T. Treatment of erectile failure with prostaglandin E1: a double-blind, placebo-controlled, dose-response study. *J Urol*. 1994;151:1530–1532.
62. Mulhall JP, Daller M, Traish AM, et al. Intracavernosal forskolin: role in management of vasculogenic impotence resistant to standard 3-agent pharmacotherapy. J Urol. 1997;158:1752–1758.
63. Lakin MM, Montague DK, Medendorp SV. Intracavernous injection therapy: Analysis of results and complications. J Urol. 1990;143:1138–1141.
64. Costabile R, Spevak M, Fishman I. Efficacy and safety of transurethral alprostadil in patients with erectile dysfunction following radical prostatectomy. J Urol. 1998;160:1325–1328.
65. Goldstein I, Lue TF, Padma-Nathan H, Rosen RC, Steers WD, Wicker PA. Oral sildenafil in the treatment of erectile dysfunction. *N Engl J Med*. 1998;338:1397–1404.
66. Licht M. Sildenafil for treating male erectile dysfunction. *Cleveland Clin J Med*. 1998;65:301–304.

67. Boolell M, Gepi-Attee S, Gingell J, Allen M. Sildenafil, a novel effective oral therapy for male erectile dysfunction. *Br J Urol.* 1996;78:257–261.
68. Zippe CD, Kedia AW, Kedia K, Nelson DR, Agarwal A. Treatment of erectile dysfunction after radical prostatectomy with sildenafil citrate (Viagra). *Urology.* 1998;52:963–966.
69. Freedman A, Hahn G, Love N. Follow-up after therapy for prostate cancer. Treating the problems and caring for the man. *Postgrad Med.* 1996;100:125–129,133–134,136.
70. van Andel G, Kurth KH. The impact of androgen deprivation therapy on health-related quality of life in asymptomatic men with lymph node positive prostate cancer. *Eur Urol.* 2003;44:209–214.
71. Garnick MB. Screening diagnosis, and management. *Ann Intern Med.* 1993;118:804–818.

Advanced Prostate Cancer: Symptom Management

BLADDER OUTLET OBSTRUCTION

Cause

- Compression of the prostatic urethra by tumor mass or enlarged lymph nodes

Signs and Symptoms of Impending Blockage[1]

- Frequency
- Urgency
- Nocturia
- Slow urinary stream

Signs and Symptoms of Blockage

- Inability to void
- Lower abdominal pain and pressure

Unrelieved, Will Result In

- Distended bladder
- Hydronephrosis
- Renal failure

Onset

- Acute vs. chronic

Treatment Options

Indwelling urinary catheter[1]
- Insert indwelling urinary drainage catheter. Placement may be difficult. Monitor for infection, bacterial colonization, bladder spasms, and chronic indwelling catheter problems.

Suprapubic catheter
- Monitor for infection, change dressing daily and as needed.

Clean intermittent self-catheterization[2, 3]
- Requires patient commitment to self-catheterize every 3–4 hours and at bedtime
- Fluid intake of 2 liters/day until 3 hours prior to bedtime; consumed in small frequent amounts throughout the day
- Include cranberry juice in diet. (See **Table 15–1** for nursing care standard.)
- Monitor residual urine.

Hormonal manipulation
- Requires 2–3 weeks of therapy before response seen[1]

Transurethral resection of the prostate (TURP)
Channel TURP

TABLE 15–1 Standard of Care for the Patient with Advanced Prostate Cancer

NURSING DIAGNOSIS: Knowledge deficit related to performance of intermittent self-catheterization

PATIENT OUTCOME: Patient/SO will be able to perform intermittent self-catheterization

NURSING INTERVENTIONS:

1. Assess pt's understanding of urinary tract anatomy and how to perform self-catheterization.

2. Use anatomic pictures or 3D models of urinary tract to teach pt location of bladder and urethra.

3. Instruct pt family in clean technique of self-catheterization.
   - Wash hands well with soap and running water and dry.
   - Gather equipment.
   - Wash penis with soap and water, rinse and dry. Retract foreskin.
   - Set up supplies.
   - A lubricant may be used to ease catheter insertion.
   - Grasp and straighten penis and lift upward while inserting catheter.
   - Completely empty bladder. Remove catheter and replace foreskin to usual position.
   - Wash and dry catheter and store in a clean plastic self-closing bag.

4. Teach pt to balance fluid consumption throughout day and not to consume large amounts of fluid at one time. Total fluid volume consumed each day should be about two liters. Fluids consumed should include cranberry juice.

5. Self-catheterization must be performed on a routine schedule of every 34 hours and at bedtime. About 350–400 mL urine should be obtained with each catheterization.

6. Symptoms of urosepsis, such as fever, chills, or change in appearance of urine, must be reported to nurse or physician. Institute appropriate antibiotic therapy as prescribed.

NURSING DIAGNOSIS: Knowledge deficit related to care of PNT

PATIENT OUTCOME: The pt/SO will be able to demonstrate care of PNT

NURSING INTERVENTIONS:

1. Assess pt/SO understanding of purpose of PNT.

2. Teach pt/SO in care of PNT. Wash hands. Cleanse around tube exit site with saline or soap and water according to policy. Pat dry. Cover exit site with dry gauze and tape securely in place.

3. Tubes must be securely taped in place at all times to avoid dislodgment.

4. Inspect exit site with each dressing change for infection (e.g., redness, change in color, or amount of drainage). Report changes to nurse or physician.

5. Empty PNT drainage bag when ½ to ⅔ full to avoid overfilling of bag.

6. Use clean technique when emptying bags to avoid contamination.

7. Monitor pt for other complications of PNT (i.e., reduced urine output from dislodgment or blockage and bleeding). Notify physician.

8. Teach pt about importance of maintaining schedule of appointments for routine catheter changes, usually every three months or as prescribed by physician.

9. Tubing must not be kinked, which would block urine flow. It must be taped to be maintained in a straight position.

TABLE 15–1 Standard of Care for the Patient with Advanced Prostate Cancer, continued

10. Flush PNT with NSS as ordered. Teach pt to prepare NSS flush and how to flush PNT.

11. Instruct patient to use leg drainage bag during day and straight drainage bag at night.

12. Instruct patient on care of drainage bags. Rinse with diluted vinegar and water (1:3), rinse well with water, and air dry or care for as per hospital policy.

NURSING DIAGNOSIS: Risk for infection related to catheters in urinary tract or urinary retention

PATIENT OUTCOME: Pt will have prompt recognition of s-s of UTI

NURSING INTERVENTIONS:

1. Assess urine and catheters for sign of infection: odor, color, purulent drainage, change in clarity, pain.

2. Monitor vital signs for infection: ↑T, ↑HR, ↑respiratory rate, ↓BP.

3. Obtain urine culture and blood cultures as ordered.

4. Administer antipyretics, antibiotics as ordered.

5. Teach pt s-s of UTI and to notify nurse or physician when s-s present.

6. Use clean technique when emptying drainage bags and doing catheter care.

7. Never raise drainage bag above level of bladder.

8. Empty drainage bag when $\frac{1}{2}$ to $\frac{2}{3}$ full.

9. Keep drainage bags off floor. Hang from bed frame.

10. Keep tubing straight to allow for drainage.

11. Teach pt to perform meatal care with soap and water and to perform twice a day when indwelling urinary catheter in place.

12. Teach pt/SO to change to straight urinary drainage bag at night and to use leg bag during day.

13. Teach patient/SO on use of good hand washing prior to catheterization, PNT care, or drainage bag changes.

NURSING DIAGNOSIS: Potential for deficit fluid volume and electrolyte imbalances from postrenal obstruction

PATIENT OUTCOME: Pt will have prompt recognition of fluid and electrolyte abnormalities

NURSING INTERVENTIONS:

1. Assess I&O; daily weights; q 2 hour vital signs.

2. Monitor fluid balance closely after placement of catheters because diuresis often occurs after obstruction relieved.

3. Monitor lab results, BUN, creatinine, electrolytes, and notify physician of abnormal results.

4. Administer IV fluids and electrolytes as ordered.

5. Monitor amount of peripheral edema.

6. Notify physician of urine output > 200 mL/hr lasting for two hours.

NURSING DIAGNOSIS: Impaired comfort related to scrotal edema

PATIENT OUTCOME: Pt will verbalize increased comfort level

NURSING INTERVENTIONS:

1. Assess amount of edema.

2. Assess level of discomfort using scale ranging from 0 to 10.

continues

TABLE 15–1 Standard of Care for the Patient with Advanced Prostate Cancer, continued

3. Elevate scrotum on folded towels placed between thighs or use towel as a supportive device by laying towel across legs and placing scrotum on top of towel. Change towel at least daily and when wet or soiled.

4. Monitor for signs of infection such as redness, drainage, pain.

5. Provide good skin care: Wash skin well and thoroughly dry twice a day and when wet.

NURSING DIAGNOSIS: Impaired comfort related to leg edema

PATIENT OUTCOME: Pt will verbalize increased comfort

NURSING INTERVENTIONS:

1. Assess severity of leg edema. Measure legs daily and record measurements. Daily weight.

2. Assess level of discomfort using a scale ranging from 0 to 10.

3. Elevate legs above heart.

4. Consider consultation to multidisciplinary lymphedema program after discussion with physician.

5. Educate pt to avoid injury to feet and skin on legs. Pt should wear clean socks and shoes at all times. Nail care should be done by a podiatrist. Skin must be inspected daily for breakage. After washing skin, lubricate with lotion.

6. Consider use of gentle exercise to reduce edema. Consult physical therapist after discussion with physician.

7. Avoid tight constrictive garments on affected leg other than compression garment.

8. Teach pt/SO to apply compression devices, garments.

NURSING DIAGNOSIS: Anticoagulation therapy for DVT

PATIENT OUTCOME: Pt will not sustain an injury from anticoagulation therapy

NURSING INTERVENTIONS:

1. Educate pt as to bleeding precautions.

2. Obtain baseline PT/INR, PTT, platelet counts as ordered and monitor results throughout therapy.

3. Obtain specimens from peripheral vein or from central venous catheter according to institutional policy.

4. Initiate heparin therapy with heparin bolus and follow with continuous infusion of heparin.

5. Institute bleeding precautions. Educate pt to avoid injury, use an electric razor and use a toothette for oral care.

6. Repeat PTT in six hours after start of heparin therapy, adjust rate as ordered, and check PTT after each infusion rate change. Report results to physician.

7. Start warfarin after heparin drip initiated.

8. Monitor pt for bleeding.

9. Monitor platelet count. If platelet count falls < 100,000 or falls quickly, notify physician and interrupt heparin infusion. Pt may be developing HITT.

10. After heparin level therapeutic, monitor daily PTT.

11. Educate pt as to use of warfarin at home and need for ongoing monitoring of PT/INR while on therapy. Educate pt on administration of SQ LMWH.

12. Consult home health nurse to monitor PT/INR at home and assess pt.

TABLE 15–1 Standard of Care for the Patient with Advanced Prostate Cancer, continued

13. Educate patient to avoid grapefruits, grapefruit juice, cranberry juice, and foods high in vitamin K. Educate patient that there are many drugs that interact with warfarin and that he should notify all health care providers that he takes warfarin.

NURSING DIAGNOSIS: Thrombocytopenia related to DIC-induced bleeding

PATIENT OUTCOME: Pt will have reduced bleeding

NURSING INTERVENTIONS:

1. Assess body system for bleeding:
   - Skin: Oozing, petechiae, ecchymoses
   - Mucous membranes of nose and mouth, rectum for bleeding
   - CNS: Neurologic checks, level of consciousness, vision changes, headache, confusion
   - Lungs: Pulse oximetry, chest pain, hemoptysis, abnormal breath sounds, cyanosis, mottling, tachypnea
   - Cardiovascular: Tachycardia, hypotension, vital sign changes, arrhythmias
   - Renal: Hematuria, oliguria, I&O, BUN, creatinine
   - Extremities: Pulses, color sensation, motor activity
   - GI tract: Bowel sounds, abdominal distention, melena, hematemesis, hematochezia
   - Any prior venipuncture site or site of injury
   - Pain level
2. Institute bleeding precautions: no IM injections, no enemas or suppositories, no aspirin or NSAIDs, no razors.
3. Use sponge toothettes for oral care.
4. Obtain and monitor lab work results.
5. Administer prescribed blood products, heparin, antibiotics, volume expanders, IV fluids, oxygen.
6. Avoid invasive procedures and venipunctures.
7. Monitor vital signs, I&O, neurologic checks q 4 hours. Avoid automated BP cuffs.
8. Elevate HOB to improve ventilation. Encourage coughing and deep breathing.
9. Turn q 2 hours to reduce pressure.
10. Monitor amount of blood loss.
11. Test urine, stool, and emesis for blood. Monitor sputum for blood.
12. Apply direct pressure to bleeding sites.
13. Consult dentist to pack bleeding gums. Provide gentle oral care, saline mouth rinses.
14. Offer pain medication.
15. Institute safety precautions, prone to fall precautions.
16. Keep pt warm: Use blankets, change wet linens and gown.
17. Perform gentle range of motion.

NURSING DIAGNOSIS: Anxiety related to disease process

PATIENT OUTCOME: Pt will have reduced anxiety

NURSING INTERVENTIONS:

1. Assess level of anxiety.
2. Consult with social worker to assist with helping pt manage anxiety.

continues

TABLE 15–1 Standard of Care for the Patient with Advanced Prostate Cancer, continued

3. Use distraction and relaxation exercises, such as music therapy and guided imagery.

4. Encourage pt verbalization. Offer support.

NURSING DIAGNOSIS: Impaired comfort related to pain in bones

PATIENT OUTCOME: Pt will verbalize adequate level of analgesia

NURSING INTERVENTIONS:

1. Assess pain using scale ranging from 0 to 10. Identify location, onset, duration, precipitating and alleviating factors. Document data on a pain assessment form. Encourage pt to keep a pain diary.

2. Administer routine and rescue analgesics, NSAIDs, and other medications for pain.

3. Administer stool softeners and laxatives to prevent narcotic-induced constipation. Educate pt to increase fluid consumption.

4. Reevaluate analgesic regimen on routine basis and titrate doses as needed.

5. Reduce dose as needed after administration of bone-seeking radionuclide, radiation therapy, or other pain-reducing therapy.

6. Educate pt as to management of pain at home.

7. Educate pt to use of heat and cold, distraction, music therapy, and other forms of pain control.

8. Consult pain management team as needed.

9. Consult with PT-OT to enhance mobility.

10. Use therapeutic mattress to reduce pain.

11. Administer zoledronic acid 4 mg in 100 ml IV fluid as a PB over 15 minutes. Dose must be adjusted for elevated creatinine levels even if the level is still within the normal range. Check electrolytes, ions, BUN, creatinine, CBC before administering. Modify dose based on serum creatinine. Run as an IV PB with saline. Flush line well before and after administration. Assess patient's level of hydration before administration. Do not administer in presence of dehydration. Monitor vital signs before administration and at end of infusion. Educate patient as to drug-related side effect profile and self-care management of side effects and when to notify nurse or physician of side effects. Instruct patient to take vitamin D (400 IU) and calcium (500 mg) daily. Baseline dental exam should be done before starting therapy.

Pt, patient; 3D, three dimensional; PNT, percutaneous nephrostomy tube; SO, significant other; NSS, normal saline solution; s-s, signs and symptoms; UTI, urinary tract infection; T, temperature; HR, heart rate; BP, blood pressure; I & O, intake and output; BUN, blood urea nitrogen; IV, intravenous; PT/INR, prothrombin time/international normalized ratio; PTT, partial thromboplastin time; HITT, heparin-induced thrombocytopenia and thrombosis; DIC, disseminated intravascular coagulation; CNS, central nervous system; GI, gastrointestinal; IM, intramuscular; NSAIDs, nonsteroidal anti-inflammatory drugs; HOB, head of bed; PT, physical therapy; OT, occupational therapy; PB, piggyback; CBC, complete blood count.

Compiled from Weber-Jones,[2] Dagler,[3] Modic et al.,[4] Gulmi et al.,[15] Humble,[16] Galindo-Ciocon,[18] Lechner,[26] Majoros and Moccia,[30] Simko and Lockhart,[31] Elzer and Houdek,[29] Schafer,[79] Nakashima et al,[101] Belcher,[45] Dressler,[49] Ibrahim et al.,[74] Saad, et al,[75] Maxwell, et al,[94] Schumacher et al.,[79] Mayer et al.,[80] Struthers et al.,[81] Schulam et al.,[99] Sullano and Ortiz,[100] Carpenito-Moyet.[97]

Source: Held-Warmkessel, J. Advanced prostate cancer: symptom management. In: Held-Warmkessel, J., ed. *Contemporary Issues in Prostate Cancer: A Nursing Perspective* (2nd ed). Jones and Bartlett Publishers, 2006, 353–391. Reprinted with permission by Jones and Bartlett Publishers.

Radiation therapy[5, 6]
- Side effects include dysuria and bowel toxicity.

Urethral stents[7–10]
- Intraurethral diameter increases to promote normal voiding.
- Suprapubic cystostomy tube may be placed preoperatively and left open to drain for 24 hours after surgery.
- Variety of stents available including woven mesh and self-expanding coils. Promote voiding in 88–100 % of patients treated. Patent several years in some patients.
- Postoperative complications—dysuria, blood clots, frequency, nocturia, urgency, transient hematuria, perineal pain. May last up to 1 month after stent placement.

Urinary tract infections—manage with antibiotics.

URETERAL OBSTRUCTION
Cause[5, 11, 12]
- Blockage of ureters by enlarged lymph nodes, trigone tumor, ureterovesical junction tumor. May be bilateral.

Signs and Symptoms
- Blocked urine flow
- Hydronephrosis
- Renal failure
- Uremia (fluid and electrolyte imbalance, acidosis, anorexia, nausea, vomiting, fatigue, altered cognition, acidosis)

Onset
- May be present for months prior to development of symptoms

Treatment
Ureteral stent placement
Percutaneous nephrostomy tube (PNT) placement[3]

Side effects/complications
- Infection, bleeding, obstruction, dislodgement; must be replaced approximately every 3 months to maintain patency. Catheter may be internalized after placement or replaced with stents.[1, 13]

Signs of impending tube failure
- Reduced urine output, urine leakage, blockage, encrustation
- Requires flushing to maintain patency and dressing changes
- See **Table 15–1**.

Hormonal therapy
Radiation therapy
Dexamethasone[14]

LEG EDEMA
Causes[16–19]
- Lymphatic or venous obstruction
- Lymph node dissection
- Low serum albumin

- Lymphedema
  - Protein-rich lymphatic fluid deposited in interstitial spaces due to lymph node metastases or removal of lymph nodes
- Venous edema
  - Blocked veins reduce blood blow to heart and increase venous pressure, which promotes loss of fluid into interstitial space.
- DVTs
- Medical conditions
- Congestive heart failure
- Heart disease
- Venous insufficiency
- Renal disease
- Aging

Diagnostic Studies

- Serum albumin level
- Bilateral venous Doppler studies
- Magnetic resonance imaging (MRI) scan of the abdomen and pelvis

Signs and Symptoms[20–23]

Venous
- Unilateral swelling (may be bilateral)
- Pain present
- Dilated veins
- Redness
- Increased warmth
- Reduced mobility
- May develop quickly

Lymphatic
- Begins distally (foot)
- Tissue soft initially but becomes hard over time
- May be disabling
- Develops more slowly

Assessment (see Table 15–2)[3, 6, 16, 20, 23, 24]

Severity Assessment[16, 25]

- Venous—use scale of 0–4 (0 = no edema; 4 = edema > 1 cm)
- Lymphedema (see **Table 15–3**)

Measurements (see Figure 15–1)

- Assess daily, at same time and location on leg. Perform measurements bilaterally; document and compare measurements to determine severity, pulses, sensory function, motor function, impact on quality of life, self-care, walking, self-esteem, and level of pain (see **Table 15–3**).[24]

Treatment

Deep vein thrombosis (DVT)
- Treatment with heparin and warfarin, vena cava filter
- Pretreatment coagulation studies—prothrombin time (PT)/international normalized ration (INR)/activated partial prothrombin time (PTT), platelet count

- Heparin
  - Dosed by intravenous (IV) bolus followed by continuous infusion
  - Action—interferes with clotting factor IX and thrombin[26]
  - PTT reassessed in 6 hours. Dose of heparin adjusted to attain a PTT 1.5–2.0 times control
  - Weight-based heparin—dose based on patient's current weight
  - Weight-based low molecular weight heparin (LMWH)—twice daily subcutaneous injections followed by warfarin beginning on day 2[26, 27]
  - When INR is 2.0–3.0, both heparin and LMWH are stopped.[20, 27]
- Warfarin
  - Warfarin therapy—INR goal is 2.0–3.0
  - Initiated after heparin or LMWH therapy
  - Action—reduces amount of vitamin K-dependent clotting factors produced[20]
  - Starting dose: 2.5–10 mg per day for 1–2 days
  - Additional doses based on PT/INR results
  - Length of therapy: 3–6 months or longer[23]

TABLE 15–2 Assessment of Leg Edema

Venous Cause	Lymphatic Cause
Is the edema unilateral or bilateral?	Has the patient had a pelvic lymphadenectomy?
Has the patient been spending more time in bed?	Has an injury occurred to the affected extremity?
Are the leg(s) warm, painful, or red?	Do either or both of the legs feel heavy?
Does the patient have a low-grade temperature?	Has the patient received large doses of radiation therapy to the affected extremity?
Are the leg veins dilated?	Does elevation of the extremity reduce the swelling?
Does the patient have symptoms of pulmonary embolus, such as chest pain, anxiety, shortness of breath?	Are the toes square in appearance?
Is a positive Homans' sign present?	Is leg tissue woody, fibrotic, or indurated?

Data compiled from Humble,[16] Cantwell-Gob,[20] Farncombe and Robertson,[24] and Creager and Dzau.[27]
Source: Held-Warmkessel, J. Advanced prostate cancer: symptom management. In: Held-Warmkessel, J., ed. *Contemporary Issues in Prostate Cancer: A Nursing Perspective* (2nd ed). Jones and Bartlett Publishers, 2006, 353–391. Reprinted with permission by Jones and Bartlett Publishers.

TABLE 15–3 Severity of Lymphedema

Difference in Leg Measurements (cm)	Severity of Lymphedema
1–1.5	Diagnosable
1.5–3	Mild
3–5	Moderate
> 5	Severe

Source: From Humble CA. Lymphedema: incidence, pathophysiology, management and nursing care. *Oncology Nursing Forum.* 1995;22:1503–1509.

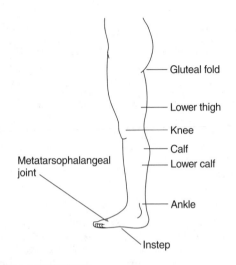

Figure 15-1. Measurement landmarks
Source: Held-Warmkessel, J. Advanced prostate cancer: symptom management. In: Held-Warmkessel, J., ed. *Contemporary Issues in Prostate Cancer: A Nursing Perspective* (2nd ed). Jones and Bartlett Publishers, 2006, 353–391. Reprinted with permission by Jones and Bartlett Publishers.

- Nursing management of DVT—see **Table 15–1**
  - Assess for bleeding from the nose, mouth, or in the urine or stool.
  - Institute bleeding precautions.
  - Monitor lab results.
- Patient education regarding injection technique, length of therapy, side effects, when to notify health care provider of side effects, side effect management, foods and diet supplements to avoid, avoiding leg massage, signs and symptoms of bleeding, need to report any bleeding, signs and symptoms of recurrent DVT, need to maintain warfarin therapy, need to maintain laboratory work schedule, use both written and oral patient education
  - Monitor for heparin-induced thrombocytopenia and thrombosis,[28, 29] pulmonary embolus (chest pain, dyspnea, shortness of breath, tachycardia, tachypnea)[30]
  - Inferior vena cava filter.

Lymphedema[24, 25, 31, 32]
  - Elevate affected extremity above heart.
  - Evaluate patient for multidisciplinary approach to lymphedema management— nursing, physical therapy, medicine. Requires time commitment from patient.
  - Components of care—skin care, education, massage, exercise, and supportive hose. Must be performed daily.
  - Medications
  - Antibiotics[24, 32]
    - Diuretics—produce volume depletion[33]

- Monitor blood pressure and for lightheadedness and dizziness.
- Coumarin—not recommended due to side effects[34, 35]

SCROTAL EDEMA[36–38]

- Cause—advanced disease and lymphedema, infection, surgery, allergic reactions, irritation, postradical prostatectomy radiation therapy, heart failure, liver failure
- Management—Keep skin folds clean and dry, elevate scrotum on clean folded towel.

DISSEMINATED INTRAVASCULAR COAGULATION (DIC)
Cause[36, 39–41]

- Triggering event stimulates clotting cascade resulting in formation of fibrin thrombi, consumption of clotting factors, and fibrinolysis
- Clots develop in small blood vessels
- Clotting factors and platelets consumed causing bleeding
- Fibrinolysis produces fibrin split products (FSP) or fibrin degradation products (FDPs) that have anticoagulation properties

Signs and Symptoms

- Acute bleeding from multiple areas including body orifices, venipuncture sites, areas of prior trauma to skin or mucous membranes, organs such as lungs, kidneys, brain, liver, or gastrointestinal tract
- Chronic DIC—few or no signs or symptoms; minor bleeding may be present from mucous membranes, skin, or GI tract[43]

Severity

- Ranges in severity from hemorrhage to ooze or with only evidence of laboratory abnormalities and without evidence of disease[42]
- Abnormal blood work/laboratory studies
- See **Table 15–4**.[36, 40, 41, 44–47]
- See **Table 15–5**.[46, 48]

Treatment

- Determination of triggering event
- Removal of triggering event
- Heparin therapy or LMWH therapy[46, 49, 50]
- Blood volume and blood product replacement—platelets, packed red blood cells, volume expanders, antithrombin concentrates
- Avoid fibrinogen-containing products that accelerate DIC[50]

Nursing Assessment (see Table 15–1)

- Complete every 4 hours and more often as needed. May be a critical care nursing challenge
- Monitor for changes in[36, 44]
  - Skin—mottling, petechiae, ecchymoses, purpura
  - Arterial—weak pulses
  - Neurologic—confusion, headaches, change in mental status, motor weakness, paralysis
  - Pulmonary—hemoptysis

TABLE 15–4 Laboratory Studies Used in the Diagnosis and Monitoring of DIC

Test	Normal Result	Value	Diagnostic of DIC
D-dimer	< 10 μcg/mL	↑	> 500 μcg/mL
FDP	10 μcg/mL	↑	> 45 μcg/mL
Antithrombin III	89–120%	↓	< 80%
Fibrinogen	200–400 mg/dL	↓	< 150–195 mg/dL
PT	12–15 seconds	↑	4–5 s above normal
Platelet count	150,000–400,000/mm[39]	↓	< 150,000–100,00/mm[39]
PTT	25–39 seconds	↑	> 60 seconds
Clotting factors		↓	

DIC, disseminated intravascular coagulation; FDP, fibrin degradation product; PT, prothrombin time; PTT, partial thromboplastin time.
Data compiled from Black & Matassarin-Jacobs,[36] Murphy-Ende,[40] Gobel,[41] Finley,[44] Belcher,[45] Bick,[46] and Gobel.[47]
Source: Held-Warmkessel, J. Advanced prostate cancer: symptom management. In: Held-Warmkessel, J., ed. *Contemporary Issues in Prostate Cancer: A Nursing Perspective* (2nd ed). Jones and Bartlett Publishers, 2006, 353–391. Reprinted with permission by Jones and Bartlett Publishers.

TABLE 15–5 New Laboratory Studies for Evaluating DIC

Test	Value
Prothrombin fragment 1 + 2	Increased
Fibrinopeptide	Increased
Platelet factor 4	Increased
Assay of thrombin precursor protein	Increased
Thrombin-antithrombin complexes	Increased

Data compiled from Bick,[46] and Van Cott & Laposata.[48]
Source: Held-Warmkessel, J. Advanced prostate cancer: symptom management. In: Held-Warmkessel, J., ed. *Contemporary Issues in Prostate Cancer: A Nursing Perspective* (2nd ed). Jones and Bartlett Publishers, 2006, 353–391. Reprinted with permission by Jones and Bartlett Publishers.

- GI—melena, hematochezia, abdominal distention, tenderness
- Renal—hematuria, oliguria, renal failure

BONE PAIN

Causes[5, 51–58]

- Local—from nearby organs
- Referred—from back, legs, abdomen
- Bone—most common etiology of pain in prostate cancer patients due to bone metastases in pelvis and spine

- Bone environment conductive to metastatic growth
- Prostate cancer cells affect osteoclast function and promote bone loss.
- Osteoblast functioning resulting in osteoblastic lesions, the most common type of bone metastases in prostate cancer
- Spinal metastases, nerve root compression with neuropathic pain
- Bone pain may be due to multiple etiologies including bone loss, new bone growth, and prostaglandins. In addition, prostaglandins may play a role in the development of bone metastases.

Diagnostic Studies

- Bone scan
- Plain radiographs

Pain Descriptors[59]

- Diffuse, ache, stab, burn
- Worse at night
- Not relieved by lying down
- Constant, intermittent, or incidental
- Joint pain

Management

Hormonal manipulation[60]
- Orchiectomy
- Antiandrogens plus luteinizing hormone-releasing hormone (LHRH) agonists

Analgesics
Nonopioids—nonsteroidal anti-inflammatory (NSAIDs) and acetaminophen [61, 62]
- Used for mild to moderate pain and for bone pain
- Monotherapy or in combination with an opioid
- Dose within usual dose range for drug to avoid toxicities[63]
- Side effects—reduced platelet aggregation, gastric ulcers, impaired renal function, dizziness, drowsiness[64]
- Avoid use in patients with liver disease or alcohol abuse.

Opioids
- Morphine, hydromorphone, oxycodone, fentanyl are appropriate for use in this patient population.[65]
- Used for moderate to severe pain
- Monotherapy or in combination with a nonopioid
- Combination products include acetaminophen plus codeine, hydrocodone, and oxycodone
- Dose within usual dose range for drug combination components to avoid toxicity
- Meperidine—not recommended for use in cancer pain
- Opioids available for administration by a variety of routes—oral, short-acting, long-acting, rectal, parenteral, topical
- Combination of short-acting and long-acting drugs may be used.
- Initiate therapy with short-acting drugs, titrate dose as needed, and convert to controlled-release formulation after good analgesia obtained with short-acting agents.
- Allow for breakthrough pain dosing on an as needed basis.
- Convert to a different analgesic if side effects are unacceptable after 3 days of therapy. New drug dose needs to be reduced by 50–66% of the equianalgesic dose of the previous agent (see **Table 15–6**).[66]

TABLE 15–6 Equianalgesic Doses of Opioid Analgesics Used for the Control of Chronic Pain

Analgesic	Oral Dose (mg)	Dose Interval
Meperidine (Demerol)	150	q2–3h
Codeine (3 tablets Tylenol No. 3)	100	q4h
Pentazocine (Talwin)	90	q4h
Hydrocodone (3 tablets/ capsules Vicodin/Lortab)	15	q4h
Morphine (MSIR, Roxanol)	15	q4h
Morphine (MS Contin, Oramorph SR)	45	q12h
Morphine (Kadian)	90	q24h
Oxycodone (2 tablets Percodan, Percocet, Roxicodone) OxyFast, 20 mg/mL, Roxicodone Intensol 20 mg/mL	10	q4h
Oxycodone (OxyContin)	30	q12h
Methadone (Dolophine)	10	q8–12h
Hydromorphone (Dilaudid)	4	q4h
Levorphanol (Levo-Dromoran)	2	q4–6h
Fentanyl (Duragesic)	NA	q72h
Oral transmucosal fentanyl citrate (Actiq)		q30 min x 2 units, max. of 4 doses/ day, begin dosage at 200 μg for all patients, for use only with narcotic-tolerant patients

DRUG, COMPANY, AND LOCATION LIST: Actiq, Anesta, Salt Lake City, UT; and Abbot, North Chicago, IL; Demerol, Talwin, Sanofi Pharmaceuticals, New York; Tylenol No. 3, Ortho-McNeil Pharmaceutical, Raritan, NJ; Vicodin, Dilaudid, Knoll Laboratories, Mt. Olive, NJ; Lortab, UCB Pharma, Inc., Smyrna, GA; MSIR, MS Contin, OxyContin, Purdue Frederick, Norwalk, VA and Purdue Pharma, Norwalk, CT; Kadian, Faulding, Raleigh, NC; Roxanol, Oramorph, Roxicet, Roxicodone Intensol, Dolophine, Roxane Laboratories, Columbus, OH; Percodan, Percocet, Endo Pharmaceuticals, Inc., Chadds Ford, PA; Levo-Dromoran, ICN Pharmaceuticals, Costa Mesa, CA; Duragesic, Janssen Pharmaceuticals, Titusville, NJ.

- Methadone—inexpensive but requires more frequent monitoring to allow for titration to balance analgesia and sedation and other toxicities
- Manage side effects
  - Constipation—see **Figure 15–2**
    - Must be expected, prevented, and managed
    - Start laxatives and stool softeners with the first dose of narcotic, and titrate to meet patient needs. Educate patient as to use of laxatives and stool softeners to manage and prevent constipation.
    - Goal is easy bowel movement every 2 days.

Subcutaneous Dose (mg)	Comments
50	Toxic metabolite. Not recommended for severe chronic pain.
60	Of limited value in severe chronic pain. Each Tylenol No. 3 tablet contains 30 mg codeine plus 325 mg acetaminophen.
30	Not recommended for severe chronic pain.
NA	Of limited value in severe chronic pain. Each Vicodin or Lortab tablet contains 5 mg hydrocodone plus 500 mg acetaminophen.
5	SC dose essentially equal to IM dose.
NA	Equianalgesic IV dose equal to 75–80% of SC dose.
NA	Rectal suppositories available. PR dose is equal to PO dose.
NA	Each Percodan or Percocet tablet contains 5 mg oxycodone plus 325 mg aspirin (Percodan), 325 mg acetaminophen (Percocet). Roxicodone tablets and OxyIR capsules contain 5 mg oxycodone alone.
NA	
5	Caution: Risk of toxicity from delayed accumulation.
1.5	SC dose essentially equal to IM dose. Equianalgesic IV dose equal to 75–80% of SC dose. Rectal suppositories available. PR dose is equal to PO dose.
1	Caution: Risk of toxicity from delayed accumulation.
NA	Duragesic fentanyl transdermal system: micrograms/hour dose of transdermal fentanyl = $\frac{1}{2} \times$ milligram/day dose of oral morphine (one 100 μg/h patch q3 days = 100 mg MS Contin PO q12h).

NA, not available; SC, subcutaneous; IM, intramuscular; IV, intravenous; PR, per rectum; PO, orally; h, hour.
Equianalgesic doses listed were obtained from a variety of sometimes conflicting studies and experiences and are meant only as guidelines for around-the-clock, standing order, analgesic therapy of chronic pain. Developed and written by M. Levy, MD, PhD. Permission to adapt format and reprint granted by M. Levy, MD. Table adapted from data published in Levy M. Pharmacologic treatment of cancer pain. N Eng J Med 1996;335:11241132. Used with permission.

- Check platelet count and white blood cell count (and ANC) prior to administering enemas or suppositories.
- Nausea—Experienced by 10–40% of patients. Antiemetics are useful.[67]
- Sedation—remove other sedating drugs from patient's drug regimen, reduce narcotic dose,[65] try another opioid, or try methylphenidate or a different neurostimulant
- Respiratory depression

External beam radiation therapy—for one or a few metastatic sites[68]
- Wide range of doses may be administered[69]
- Effective in reducing pain in 75% of treated patients[70]

Constipation is a major side effect of opiates used in the treatment of pain.
Using this algorithm may help prevent this side effect and promote
compliance to the pain management regimen.

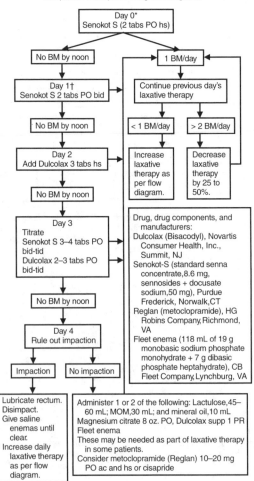

Figure 15-2. Recommended laxative therapy for cancer-associated constipation
* First day of opioid analgesia, no preexisting constipation.
†Start here if daily oral morphine equivalent ≥ 120 mg.
tabs, tablets; PO, per os; PR, per rectum; hs, bedtime; BM, bowel movement; ac, before
meals; am, morning; bid, twice a day; tid, three times a day; supp, suppository.
Sources: Adapted from data published in Levy MH. Constipation and diarrhea in cancer patients. *Cancer Bulletin* 1991;43:417. Adapted by M. Levy, P. Kedziera, and J. Koss. Used with
permission of M. Levy, MD, PhD, and *Cancer Bulletin.*

Systemic radionuclides—strontium-89 and samarium-153
- Monitor CBC and differential
- Delivers radiation therapy to metastatic bone tumors[71]
- Useful for multiple bony metastatic sites with small tumors more sensitive[68]
- About 80% of patients respond.[72]
- Bone pain flare may occur after treatment.
- Reduction in narcotic doses may be possible after pain subsides.

Nursing Assessment
- Use an assessment tool (see **Figure 15–3**).
- Determine impact of pain on quality of life, activities of daily living, impact on patient and family, and self-image.[78]
- Patient and family education—drug name, dose, route, and frequency; self-management of constipation and other side effects. Address potential concerns about addiction, dependence, and tolerance.
- Encourage use of pain diary.[79]
- Therapy may include a combination of nonopioid, opioid, and adjuvant drugs.[80]
- Nonpharmacologic interventions—heat,[80] therapeutic mattresses, assistive devices for moving, physical therapy, occupational therapy[81]

SPINAL CORD COMPRESSION (SCC)
- Serious complication of metastatic prostate cancer requiring emergency intervention to avoid complications and disability
- If back pain is present in a patient with prostate cancer, a workup for SCC should commence immediately.
- Emergency diagnosis and treatment are required to prevent paralysis and additional disability.

Cause
- Spinal metastases involving vertebral body or neural arch;[82] multiple areas may affected and may recur at previously treated site.

Location
- Thoracic spine, lumbosacral spine[83]

Signs and Symptoms
- Back pain that may radiate to legs due to pressure on nerves; muscle weakness, and sensory loss in arms, legs, or both; sensation of being squeezed around chest, trunk, or abdomen
- Autonomic nervous system changes—change in bowel or bladder function (see **Table 15–7**).

Diagnostic Studies[84–85]
- Performed emergently—plain radiographs, bone scan, MRI (best study), or computed axial tomogram (CAT) scan with myelogram

Treatment
- Dexamethasone—wide range of doses used, higher doses may be better at improving outcomes[86]
  - Monitor for side effects
  - Monitor blood sugars
  - Loading dose administered IV followed by q6h dosing[5, 87, 88]
  - Switch to oral dosing after patient is stable.
  - Administer with histamine-2 blocker or PPI

Initial Pain Assessment Tool

Date ______

Patient's Name ______________________ Age _____ Room _____

Diagnosis ____________________ Physician ____________________

Nurse ____________________

1. LOCATION: Patient or nurse mark drawing.

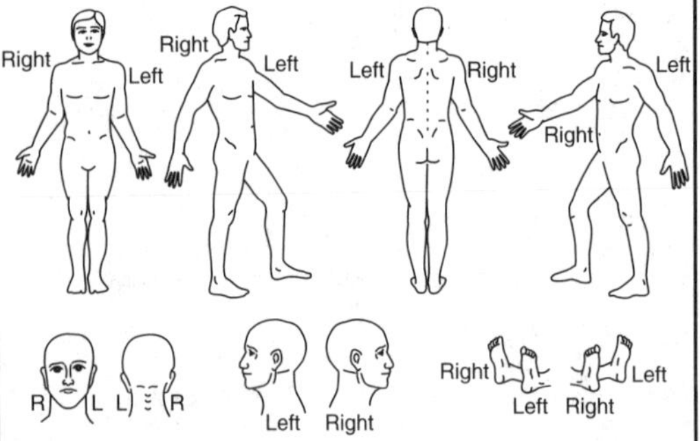

2. INTENSITY: Patient rates the pain. Scale used ____________

   Present: ____________
   Worst pain gets: ____________
   Best pain gets: ____________
   Acceptable level of pain: ____________

3. QUALITY: (Use patient's own words, e.g., prick, ache, burn, throb, pull, sharp) ____________

4. ONSET, DURATION, VARIATIONS, RHYTHMS: ____________

5. MANNER OF EXPRESSING PAIN: ____________

6. WHAT RELIEVES THE PAIN? ____________

7. WHAT CAUSES OR INCREASES THE PAIN? ____________

8. EFFECTS OF PAIN: (Note decreased function, decreased quality of life.) ____________

   Accompanying symptoms (e.g., nausea) ____________
   Sleep ____________
   Appetite ____________
   Physical activity ____________
   Relationship with others (e.g., irritability) ____________
   Emotions (e.g., anger, suicidal, crying) ____________
   Concentration ____________
   Other ____________

9. OTHER COMMENTS: ____________

10. PLAN: ____________

FIGURE 15-3 Initial pain assessment tool

Source: Reprinted from *Pain: Clinical Manual,* McCaffery M, Pasero C, p. 60. Copyright 1999, with permission from Elsevier.

- Radiation therapy—20–30 Gy[85]
- Neurosurgery

Nursing Management [84, 88, 90–97]

- Dependent on severity of paralysis
- Neurologic assessments—sensory, motor, and autonomic
- Pain management
- Assess impact on quality of life
- Safety—mandatory bed rest until spinal stability determined by physician
- Patient education—signs and symptoms of SCC; once treated, SCC may recur; self-care management of side effects and complications of SCC what symptoms and signs to report to physician
- Physical therapy consult for reconditioning
- Social service consult for support and discharge planning
- Ongoing assessment and monitoring
- Cervical (Philadelphia) collars for cervical spine lesions
- Braces may be appropriate for other spine lesions[98]
- See **Table 15–8**

TABLE 15–7 Types of Pain Associated with Spinal Cord Compression

Location	Description
Local	Tenderness at site of tumor
	Progresses from mild to severe
	Present in 95% of patients
	Constant
	Increases with recumbent position, leg raising
	Increases with coughing and sneezing
	Increases at night
Radicular	Tight band around area of body at level of cord compression
	Spreads to legs
	Dermatomal distribution
	Increases with coughing, sneezing
	Unilateral with cervical or lumbar lesions
Referred	Poorly localized
	Described as burning, shooting; paresthesias

Data compiled from Surya and Provent,[5] Osborn et al.,[82] Wilkes,[84] Weinstein,[85] and Faul and Flickinger.[89]

Source: Held-Warmkessel, J. Advanced prostate cancer: symptom management. In: Held-Warmkessel, J., ed. *Contemporary Issues in Prostate Cancer: A Nursing Perspective* (2nd ed). Jones and Bartlett Publishers, 2006, 353–391. Reprinted with permission by Jones and Bartlett Publishers.

TABLE 15–8 Nursing Care Standard for Patients with SCC

NURSING DIAGNOSIS: Knowledge deficit related to the etiology and treatment of SCC

DESIRED PATIENT OUTCOME: Pt will verbalize the s-s of SCC. Pt immediately will notify the physician of any symptoms of SCC.

NURSING INTERVENTIONS:

1. Assess pt/SO understanding of etiology, diagnosis, and treatment of SCC.

2. Educate pt/SO about cause, diagnostic workup, treatment goals, and treatment of SCC.

3. Educate prostate cancer patients about s-s of SCC and need for prompt medical intervention. High-risk patients have > 20 metastatic sites on bone scan or have been on androgen deprivation therapy.

   • Back pain (early sign)

   • Pain produced by percussion over spine

   • Pain radiating from back along dermatome to chest, abdomen, groin, legs, or buttock

   • Change in motor functioning and ability to walk

   • Decreased sensation in extremities

   • Loss of muscle tone

   • Constipation

   • Urinary retention

   • Loss of bowel–bladder continence (late sign)

DESIRED PATIENT OUTCOME: Pt/SO will verbalize understanding of SCC-related complications and methods used to manage complications.

NURSING INTERVENTIONS:

1. Educate pt/SO about self-care management of SCC-related complications and treatment-related side effects.

   • Radiation therapy—skin care (with high doses of radiation), bone marrow depression, diarrhea (L-spine), esophagitis (cervical, thoracic spine), nausea

   • Pressure sores and their prevention

   • Bowel–bladder continence regimen

   • Safety

   • Weakness-fatigue; rest intervals between periods of activity; afternoon naps

   • Care of bowel-bladder continence devices and use of appropriate medications and procedures

   • Surgery: Routine pre- and post-op care (e.g., pulmonary hygiene, pain management, log rolling)

   • Possible complications (e.g., infection, bleeding, pneumonia, deep vein thrombosis)

   • Steroids: take with food or antacids; monitor for s-s of side effects.

NURSING DIAGNOSIS: Impaired physical mobility related to SCC

DESIRED PATIENT OUTCOME: Pt will not experience additional deterioration of motor or sensory function.

NURSING INTERVENTIONS:

1. Assess pt's neurologic status, sensory perception, ability to walk or bear weight on legs, and ability to move around in bed and from side to side.

TABLE 15–8 Nursing Care Standard for Patients with SCC, continued

2. Document neurologic status every shift or as prescribed; may be as frequent as every 2 hours for first three days; continued until stable and then as needed. Notify physician of changes in patient's neurologic status.

3. Consult physical therapy personnel to initiate rehabilitation program as soon as medical condition stabilizes.

4. Encourage pt to change position at least every 2 hours, if appropriate.

5. Perform range-of-motion exercises on affected extremities; encourage pt to practice exercises as prescribed by physical therapist.

6. Consult occupational therapist to initiate program for assisting pt in resuming independent activities of daily living.

7. Consider pt's spine to be unstable until diagnostic studies are completed, and maintain strict bed rest until the pt is allowed out of bed.

8. Have pt use brace when out of bed to stabilize spine.

9. Have patient with a cervical lesion wear cervical collar at all times; avoid turning neck and neck rotation.

10. Use footdrop protection devices.

NURSING DIAGNOSIS: Risk for impaired skin integrity related to altered bowel or urinary elimination or impaired immobility

DESIRED PATIENT OUTCOME: Pt will be free from pressure sores. Pt will have a bowel movement only after administration of suppository. Pt will not become constipated or experience impaction. Pt will be continent of bowel all other times. Pt will not experience bladder incontinence.

NURSING INTERVENTIONS:

1. Assess integrity of skin every shift and as needed; pay particular attention to skin under braces and cervical collar.

2. Assess bowel–bladder continence, for bladder distention, and for bowel sounds.

3. Turn pt on routine schedule; use over-bed trapeze to allow for use of upper motor muscles; use special mattress to reduce risk of pressure sores, if appropriate.

4. Initiate bowel training regimen if pt is incontinent of bowel; give stool softener daily; start bisacodyl suppository M-W-F in morning after breakfast. If pt is constipated, begin routine laxatives and stool softeners at bedtime. Titrate dose to achieve goal of easy bowel movement every other day.

5. If pt experiences urinary incontinence, apply condom catheter or insert indwelling urinary catheter. If pt experiences urinary retention, insert indwelling urinary catheter or initiate program of intermittent straight catheterization.

6. Encourage intake of oral fluids (for pts on intermittent straight catheterization regimens; hold fluids after 8 pm)

7. Monitor pt for signs of paralytic ileus and impaction.

8. Encourage high-fiber diet and consumption of prunes, prune juice, and large volumes of fluids (3 L/day).

NURSING DIAGNOSIS: Risk for infection related to surgical intervention

DESIRED PATIENT OUTCOME: Pt's incision will be clean and intact. Pt's wounds will heal without complication. Pt will be free from wound infection.

continues

TABLE 15–8 Nursing Care Standard for Patients with SCC, continued

NURSING INTERVENTIONS:

1. Assess wound for signs of infection daily.

2. Assess wound for delayed healing or dehiscence resulting from radiation therapy (radiation portal usually will include most of wound. New procedures require an abdominal approach or are minimally invasive and use small incisions for placement of scopes or injection of bone cement.)

3. Change dressing at least daily.

4. Monitor pt for cerebrospinal fluid leak and signs of meningitis.

5. Take vital signs every 4 hours for 24 hours and then every shift and as needed or as per facility policy.

6. Culture wound if signs of infection are present.

7. Encourage high-protein, high-calorie diet.

NURSING DIAGNOSIS: Impaired comfort

DESIRED PATIENT OUTCOME: Pt will experience minimal pain.

NURSING INTERVENTIONS:

1. Assess quantity and quality of pain, and reassess at least every shift.

2. Administer narcotics with NSAIDs, if appropriate, on a routine and prn basis.

3. Consult with physician if pt is receiving inadequate analgesia from prescribed medication(s).

4. Administer dexamethasone, as prescribed.

5. Turn pt using log-rolling technique.

6. Keep pt's body in proper alignment.

7. Encourage use of relaxation, imagery, and diversional activity.

8. Premedicate before radiation therapy treatments and before other painful activities.

9. Administer prescribed zoledronic acid. (See Table 15-1.)

10. Utilize heat or cold applications as adjuvants to pain medications.

NURSING DIAGNOSIS: High risk for ineffective breathing pattern related to general anesthesia or to high cervical spine lesions

DESIRED PATIENT OUTCOME: Pt will maintain normal breathing pattern.

NURSING INTERVENTIONS:

1. Assess respiration (including rate and depth), cough, presence of rales, or wheezing at least daily.

2. Encourage pt to cough, deep breathe, and move around in bed every hour.

3. Get pt out of bed every shift, if not contraindicated by medical condition or unstable spine.

4. Monitor for systemic signs and symptoms of infection; culture sputum, if appropriate, and notify physician.

5. Suction as needed.

6. Take routine postoperative vital signs.

7. Consult respiratory therapy personnel for chest physical therapy and incentive spirometry.

NURSING DIAGNOSIS: Deep vein thrombosis

DESIRED PATIENT OUTCOME: Pt will be free from deep vein thrombosis.

TABLE 15-8 Nursing Care Standard for Patients with SCC, continued

NURSING INTERVENTIONS:

1. Assess pt for presence of Homans' sign, calf pain, tenderness, redness, and edema at least once a shift and before performing range-of-motion exercises.

2. Perform range-of-motion exercises with morning and evening care and with turning.

3. Notify physician of presence of signs and symptoms of deep vein thrombosis.

4. Apply antiembolic stockings or intermittent compression stockings as prescribed.

NURSING DIAGNOSIS: Disturbed sensory perception

DESIRED PATIENT OUTCOME: Pt will be free from injury.

NURSING INTERVENTIONS:

1. Assess pt for loss of pain and temperature sensation and for sensory deficits, paresthesias, impaired motor status (gait, coordination, range of motion), and impaired ability to perform activities of daily living.

2. Assess pt's environment for hazards that obstruct mobility (e.g., furniture obstructing pathways, loose objects, wet spots on floor).

3. Protect pt from thermal and other types of injury.

4. Keep pt on bed rest if spine is unstable.

5. Keep cervical collar intact if pt has cervical lesion.

6. Have pt use brace when out of bed.

7. Log roll to avoid twisting spine.

8. Avoid stress or pressure to bones at risk of fracture.

9. Use towels, pillows, and blankets to position pt every 2 hours.

10. Keep head of postop pt's bed at 30° angle.

11. Keep upper side rails elevated to aide patient while turning and repositioning and call bell light and personal items in reach. Consider use of overbed trapeze to aide with repositioning.

NURSING DIAGNOSIS: Risk for ineffective coping related to living with the risk of an oncologic emergency and with anxiety, depression, residual disability, loss of control, or threat of loss of life

DESIRED PATIENT OUTCOME: Pt will be helped to adapt to diagnosis of SCC, its accompanying self-care deficits, and potential loss of life.

NURSING INTERVENTIONS:

1. Assess pt's type and level of altered coping.

2. Include family–SO in assessment, planning, and implementation of care plan.

3. Assist pt in developing realistic and achievable short-term goals.

4. Offer support and active listening.

5. Consult with oncology social worker to assist with counseling and discharge planning and referrals to hospice, visiting nurse, or rehabilitation center.

6. Consult with psychiatry or psychiatric liaison nurse, if appropriate.

7. Consider use of antianxiety or antidepressant medications prn.

NURSING DIAGNOSIS: Risk for ineffective sexuality patterns related to motor deficits, psychological distress, or family disruption.

DESIRED PATIENT OUTCOME: Pt will be helped to adapt to altered sexuality.

continues

TABLE 15–8 Nursing Care Standard for Patients with SCC, continued

NURSING INTERVENTIONS:

1. Assess importance of sexual activity to pt's quality of life.

2. Assess changes in sexual function caused by SCC and cancer diagnosis.

3. Educate pt about relationship between SCC and altered sexual functioning.

4. Discuss intimacy concerns and alternate forms of sexual expression (e.g., holding, touching, kissing, cuddling).

5. Consult with or refer to sexual rehabilitation counselor, if appropriate.

SCC, spinal cord compression; pt, patient; SO, significant other; s-s, signs-symptoms; pre-op, preoperative; post-op, postoperative; M-W-F, Monday-Wednesday-Friday; NSAIDs, non-steroidal anti-inflammatory drugs; PRN, as occasion requires.

Based on information Wilkes,[84] Lablaw et al.,[88] Klimo and Schmidt.,[90] Halpin, et al.,[91] Bayley, et al.,[92] Sitton,[93] Shelton,[94] Grandt,[95] Forster,[96] and Carpenito-Moyet.[97]

Source: Adapted, revised, and updated 2004 from Held JL and Peahota A. Nursing care of the patient with spinal cord compression. *Oncology Nursing Forum.* 1993;20:15071516. Used with permission. Copyright Oncology Nursing Society.

References

1. Arrison DP, Hirshberg SJ, Greenberg RE. Urologic issues of palliative care. In: Berger A, Portenoy RK, Weissman DE, eds. *Principles and Practice of Palliative Care and Supportive Oncology.* 2nd ed. Philadelphia, Pa: Lippincott Williams & Wilkins; 2002:463–476.

2. Weber-Jones JE. Performing clean intermittent self-catheterization. *Nursing '91.* 1991;21:56–59.

3. Degler MA. Assessment of renal and urinary tract function. In: Smeltzer SC, Bare BG, eds. *Brunner & Suddarth's Textbook of Medical-Surgical Nursing.* 10th ed. Philadelphia, Pa: Lippincott Williams & Wilkins; 2004: 1251–1308.

4. Modic MB, Calabrese DA, Stokes RA, et al. Renal and urologic care. In: *Nursing Procedures.* 3rd ed. Springhouse, Pa: Springhouse; 2000: 582–619.

5. Surya BV, Provent JA. Manifestations of advanced prostate cancer: prognosis and treatment. *J Urol.* 1989;142:921–928.

6. Wells P, Hoskin PJ, Towler J, et al. The effect of radiotherapy on ureteral obstruction from carcinoma of the prostate. *Br J Urol.* 1996;78:752–755.

7. Gottfried HW, Gnann R, Brandle E, et al. Treatment of high-risk patients with sub-vesical obstruction from advanced prostate cancer using a thermo-sensitive mesh stent. *Br J Urol.* 1997;80:623–627.

8. Yachia D, Aridogan IA. The use of a removable stent in patients with prostate cancer and obstruction. *J Urol.* 1996;155:1956–1958.

9. Guazzoni G, Montorsi F, Bergamaschi F, et al. Prostatic UroLume Wallstent for urinary retention due to advanced prostate cancer: a 1-year follow up study. *J Urol.* 1994;152:1530–1532.

10. Perry MJA, Roodhouse AJ, Gidlow AB, et al. Thermo-expandable intraprostatic stents in bladder outlet obstruction: an 8-year study. *BJU Int.* 2002: 216–223.

11. Saitoh H, Yoshida K, Uchijima Y, et al. Two different lymph node metastatic patterns of a prostatic cancer. *Cancer.* 1990;65:1843–1846.

12. O'Reilly PH. The effect of prostatic obstruction on the upper urinary tract. In: Fitzpatrick JM, Krane RJ, eds. *The Prostate.* Edinburgh, UK: Churchill Livingstone; 1989:111–118.

13. Tekin MI, Aytekin C, Aygun C, et al. Covered metallic ureteral stent in the management of malignant ureteral obstruction: preliminary results. *Urology.* 2001;58:919–923.

14. Hamdy FC, Williams JL. Use of dexamethasone for ureteric obstruction in advanced prostate cancer: percutaneous nephrostomies can be avoided. *Br J Urol.* 1995;75:782–785.

15. Gulmi FA, Felsen D, Vaughan ED. Pathophysiology of urinary tract obstruction. In: Walsh PC, Retik AB, Vaughan ED, et al, eds. *Campbell's Urology.* 8th ed. Philadelphia, Pa: Saunders; 2002:411–462.

16. Humble CA. Lymphedema: incidence, pathophysiology, management and nursing care. *Oncol Nurs Forum.* 1995;22:1503–1509.

17. Ruschhaupt WF III. The swollen limb. In: Young JR, Graor RA, Olin JW, Bartholomew JR, eds. *Peripheral Vascular Diseases.* St. Louis, Mo: Mosby-Yearbook; 1991:639–650.

18. Ciocon J, Fernandez B, Ciocon DG. Leg edema: clinical clues to the differential diagnosis. *Geriatrics.* 1993;48;34–45.

19. Galindo-Ciocon D. Nursing care of elders with leg edema. *J Gerontol Nurs.* 1995;21:7–11.

20. Cantwell-Gob K. Assessment and management of patients with vascular disorders and problems of peripheral circulation. In: Smeltzer SC, Bare BG, eds. *Brunner & Suddarth's Textbook of Medical-Surgical Nursing.* 10th ed. Philadelphia, Pa: Lippincott Williams & Wilkins; 2004:815–853.

21. Van Gerpen R, Mast ME. Thromboembolic disorders in cancer. *Clin J Oncol Nurs.* 2004;8:289–299.

22. Wyatt LE, Miller TA. Lymphedema and tumors of the lymphatics. In: Moore WS, ed. *Vascular Surgery: A Comprehensive Review.* Philadelphia, Pa: WB Saunders; 2002:860–873.

23. Creager MA, Dzau VJ. Vascular diseases of the extremities. In: Braunwald E, Fauci AS, Kasper DL, et al, eds. *Harrison's Principles and Practice of Internal Medicine.* 15th ed. New York: McGraw Hill; 2001:1434–1442.

24. Farncombe ML, Robertson ED. Lymphedema. In: Berger A, Portenoy RK, Weissman DE, eds. *Principles and Practice of Palliative Care and Supportive Oncology.* 2nd ed. Philadelphia, Pa: Lippincott Williams & Wilkins; 2002:333–343.

25. Pappas CJ, O'Donell TF. Long-term results of compression treatment for lymphedema. *J Vasc Surg.* 1992;16:555–564.

26. Lechner DL. Sizing up your patients for heparin therapy. *Nursing '98.* 1998;28:36–41.

27. Levine M, Gent M, Hirsh J, et al. A comparison of low-molecular-weight heparin administration primarily at home with unfractionated heparin administered in the hospital for proximal deep vein thrombosis. *N Engl J Med.* 1996;334:677–681.

28. Simko LC, Lockhart JS. Heparin-induced thrombocytopenia and thrombosis. *Nursing '96.* 1996;26:33.

29. Elzer R, Houdek DL. Case managing heparin-induced thrombocytopenia. *Clin Nurse Spec.* 1998;12:238–243.

30. Majoros KA, Moccia, JM. Pulmonary embolus. *Nursing '96.* 1996;26:27–31.

31. Smith JK. Oncology nursing in lymphedema management. *Innov Breast Cancer Care.* 1998;3:82–87.

32. Cheville AL, McGarvey CL, Petrek JA, et al. Lymphedema management. *Sem Radiat Oncol.* 2003;13:290–301.

33. Hardy JR. Lymphedema-prevention rather than cure. *Ann Oncol.* 1991;2:532–533.

34. Casley-Smith JR, Morgan RG, Piller NB. Treatment of lymphedema of the arms and legs with 5,6-benzo-[a]-pyrone. *N Engl J Med.* 1993;329:1158–1163.

35. Loprinzi CL, Kugler JW, Sloan JA, et al. Lack of effect of coumarin in women with lymphedema after treatment for breast cancer. *N Engl J Med*. 1999;340:346–350.

36. Black JM, Matassarin-Jacobs E, eds. *Medical-Surgical Nursing: Clinical Management for Continuity of Care*. 5th ed. Philadelphia, Pa: WB Saunders; 1997:1377–1386,1397–1443,1447–1579,2343–2385.

37. Grainger AJ, Hide IG, Elliott ST. The ultrasound appearances of scrotal oedema. *Eur J Ultrasound*. 1998;8:33–37.

38. Petrovich Z, Lieskovsky G, Langholz B, et al. Radiotherapy following radical prostatectomy in patients with adenocarcinomas of the prostate. *Int J Radiat Oncol Biol Phys*. 1991;21:949–954.

39. Myers J. Oncologic complications. In: Otto SE, ed. *Oncology Nursing*. 4th ed. St. Louis, Mo: Mosby; 2001:498–581.

40. Murphy-Ende K. Disseminated intravascular coagulation. In: Chernecky CC, Berger BJ, eds. *Advanced and Critical Care Oncology Nursing*. Philadelphia, Pa: WB Saunders; 1998:119–139.

41. Goble BH. Disseminated intravascular coagulation. In: Yarbro CH, Frogge MH, Goodman M, et al, eds. *Cancer Nursing: Principles and Practice*. 5th ed. Sudbury, Mass: Jones and Bartlett; 2000:869–875.

42. de la Fouchardiere C, Flechon A, Droz J-P. Coagulopathy in prostate cancer. *Neth J Med*. 2003;61:347–354.

43. Goble BH. Bleeding disorders. In: Groenwald SL, Frogge MH, Goodman M, et al, eds. *Cancer Nursing: Principles and Practice*. 4th ed. Sudbury, Mass: Jones and Bartlett; 1997:604–639.

44. Finley JP. Disseminated intravascular coagulation (DIC). In: Ziegfeld CR, Lubejko BG, Shelton BK, eds. *Oncology Fact Finder: Manual of Cancer Nursing*. Philadelphia, Pa: Lippincott-Raven; 1998:436–440.

45. Belcher AE. Hematolymphatic system. In: Thompson JM, McFarland GK, Hirsch JE, et al, eds. *Mosby's Clinical Nursing*. 5th ed. St. Louis, Mo: Mosby; 2002:1151–1179.

46. Bick RL. Disseminated intravascular coagulation: current concepts of etiology, pathophysiology, diagnosis and treatment. *Hematol Oncol Clin N Am*. 2003;17:149–176.

47. Gobel BH. Disseminated intravascular coagulation. *Semin Oncol Nurs*. 1999;15:174–182.

48. Van Cott EM, Laposata M. Caogulation. In: Jacobs DS, Oxley DK, DeMott WR, eds. *Laboratory Test Handbook*. 5th ed. Hudson, Ohio: Lexi-Comp, Inc; 2001:327–358.

49. Dressler DK. DIC: coping with a coagulation crisis. *Nursing*. 2004;34:58–62.

50. Bick RL. Disseminated intravascular coagulation. *Med Clin North Am*. 1994;78: 511–543.

51. Payne R. Pain management in the patient with prostate cancer. *Cancer*. 1993;71:1131–1137.

52. Esper PS, Pienta, KJ. Supportive care in the patient with hormone refractory prostate cancer. *Semin Urol Oncol*. 1997;15:56–64.

53. Mundy GR. Mechanisms of bone metastases. *Cancer*. 1997;80:1546–1556.

54. Berruti A, Dogliotti L, Tucci M, et al. Metabolic bone disease induced by prostate cancer: rationale for use of bisphosphonates. *J Urol*. 2001 166:2023–2031.

55. Goltzman D. Mechanisms of the development of osteoblastic metastases. *Cancer*. 1997;80:1581–1587.

56. Berger AM, Koprowski C. Bone pain: assessment and management. In: Berger AM, Portenoy RK, Weissman DE, eds. *Principles and Practice of Palliative Care and Supportive Oncology*. 2nd ed. Philadelphia, Pa: Lippincott Williams & Wilkins; 2002:53–57.

57. Fulfaro F, Casuccio A, Ticozzi C, Ripamonti C. The role of bisphosphonates in the treatment of painful metastatic bone disease: a review of phase III trials. *Pain.* 1998;78:157–169.
58. Payne R. Mechanisms and management of bone pain. *Cancer.* 1997;80:1608–1613.
59. Coleman RE. Skeletal complications of malignancy. *Cancer.* 1997;80:1588–1594.
60. Taub M, Begas A, Love, N. Advanced prostate cancer: endocrine therapies and palliative measures. *Postgrad Med.* 1996;100:139–154.
61. Eisenberg E, Berkey CS, Carr DB, et al. Efficacy and safety of nonsteroidal antiinflammatory drugs for cancer pain: a meta-analysis. *J Clin Oncol.* 1994;12:2756–2765.
62. American Pain Society. *Principles of Analgesic Use in the Treatment of Acute Pain and Cancer Pain.* Glenview, Ill: American Pain Society; 2003.
63. World Health Organization Expert Committee. *Cancer Pain Relief and Palliative Care.* Geneva, Switzerland: World Health Organization; 1992.
64. McCaffery M, Portenoy RK. Nonopioids: acetaminophen and nonsteroidal antiinflammatory drugs (NSAIDs). In: McCaffery M, Pasero C, eds. *Pain: Clinical Manual.* 2nd ed. St. Louis, Mo: CV Mosby; 1999:129–160.
65. Cherney NI, Foley KM. Management of pain associated with prostate cancer. In: Raghavan D, Leibel SA, Scher HI, Lange P, eds. *Principles and Practice of Genitourinary Oncology.* Philadelphia, Pa: Lippincott-Raven; 1997:613–627.
66. Coyle N, Cherny N, Portenoy RK. Pharmacologic management of cancer pain. In: McGuire D, Yarbro C, Ferrell BR, eds. *Cancer Pain Management.* 2nd ed. Sudbury, Mass: Jones and Bartlett; 1995:89–130.
67. Campora E, Merlini L, Pace M, et al. The incidence of narcotic induced emesis. *J Pain Symptom Manage.* 1991;6:428–430
68. Brown HK, Healey JH. Metastatic cancer to the bone. In: DeVita VT, Hellman S, Rosenberg SA, eds. *Cancer: Principle and Practice of Oncology.* 6th ed. Philadelphia, Pa: Lippincott Williams & Wilkins; 2001:2713–2729.
69. Catton CN, Gospodarowicz MK. Palliative radiotherapy in prostate cancer. *Semin Urol Oncol.* 1997;15:65–72.
70. Porter AT, Fontanesi J. Palliative irradiation for bone metastases: a new paradigm [editorial]. *Int J Radiat Oncol Biol Phys.* 1994;29:1199–1200.
71. Altman GB, Lee CA. Strontium-89 for treatment of painful bone metastases from prostate cancer. *Oncol Nurs Forum.* 1996;23:523–527.
72. Robinson RG, Preston DF, Schiefelbein M, Baxter KG. Strontium-89 therapy for the palliation of pain due to osseous metastases. *JAMA.* 1995;274:420–424.
73. Morris MJ, Scher HI. Clinical approaches to osseous metastases in prostate cancer. *Oncologist.* 2003;8:161–173.
74. Ibrahim A, Scher N, Williams G, et al. Approval summary for zoledronic acid for treatment of multiple myeloma and cancer bone metastases. *Clin Ca Res.* 2003;9:2394–2399.
75. Saad F, Gleason DM, Murray R, et al. A randomized, placebo-controlled trial of zoledronic acid in patients with hormone-refractory prostate carcinoma. *J Natl Ca Institute.* 2002;94:1458–1468.
76. Saad F, Gleason DM, Murray R, et al. Long-term efficacy of zoledronic acid for the prevention of skeletal complications in patients with metastatic hormone-refractory prostate cancer. *J Nat Cancer Inst.* 2004;96:879–882.
77. Novartis Oncology. Zometa prescribing information. Novartis. 2002.
78. Iwamoto R. Men and pain. *Dev Supportive Cancer Care.* 1997;1:66–68.
79. Schumacher KL, Koresawa S, West C, et al. The usefulness of a daily pain management diary for outpatients with cancer-related pain. *Oncol Nurs Forum.* 2002;29:1304–1313.

80. Mayer DK, Struthers C, Fisher G. Bone metastases: Part II: Nursing management. *Clin J Oncol Nurs.* 1997;1:37–44.

81. Struthers C, Mayer D, Fisher G. Nursing management of the patient with bone metastases. *Semin Oncol Nurs.* 1998;14:199–209.

82. Osborn JL, Getzenberg RH, Trump DL. Spinal cord compression in prostate cancer. *J Neurol Oncol.* 1995;23:135–147.

83. Rosenthal MA, Raghavan RD, Leicester J, et al. Spinal cord compression in prostate cancer. A 10-year experience. *Br J Urol.* 1992;69:530–533.

84. Wilkes GM. Spinal cord compression. In: Yarbro CH, Frogge MH, Goodman M, eds. *Cancer Symptom Management.* 3rd ed. Boston, Mass: Jones and Bartlett; 2004:359–371.

85. Weinstein SM. Management of spinal cord and cauda equine compression. In: Berger A, Portenoy RK, Weissman DE, eds. *Principles and Practice of Palliative Care and Supportive Oncology.* 2nd ed. Philadelphia, Pa: Lippincott Williams & Wilkins; 2002:532–543.

86. Sorensen S, Helweg-Larsen S, Mouridsen H, et al. Effect of high-dose dexamethasone in carcinomatous metastatic spinal cord compression treated with radiotherapy: a randomised trial. *Eur J Cancer.* 1994;1:22–27.

87. Grossman SA, Lossignol D. Diagnosis and treatment of epidural metastases. *Oncology.* 1990;4:47–52.

88. Loblaw DA, Laperrier NJ. Emergent treatment of malignant extradural spinal cord compression: an evidence-based guide. *J Clin Oncol.* 1998;16:1613–1624.

89. Faul CM, Flickinger JC. The use of radiation in the management of spinal metastases. *J Neurol Oncol.* 1995;23:149–161.

90. Klimo P, Schmidt MH. Surgical management of spinal metastases. *Oncologist.* 2004;9:188–196.

91. Halpin RJ, Bendok BR, Liu JC. Minimally invasive treatments for spinal metastases: vertebroplasty, kyphoplasty, and radiofrequency ablation. *J Support Oncol.* 2004;2:339–351.

92. Bayley A, Milosevic M, Blend R, et al. A prospective study of factors predicting clinically occult spinal cord compression in patients with metastatic prostate carcinoma. *Cancer.* 2001;92:303–310.

93. Sitton E. Central nervous system metastases. *Semin Oncol Nurs.* 1998;14:210–219.

94. Shelton BK. Spinal cord compression. In: Ziegfeld CR, Lubejko BG, Shelton BK, eds. *Manual of Cancer Nursing.* Philadelphia, Pa: Lippincott; 1998:410–419.

95. Grandt NC. Spinal cord compression. In: Camp-Sorrell D, Hawkins RA, eds. *Clinical Manual for the Oncology Advanced Practice Nurse.* Pittsburgh, Pa: Oncology Nursing Press, Inc; 2000:799–803.

96. Forster DA. Spinal cord compression. In: Chernecky CC, Berger BJ, eds. *Advances and Critical Care Oncology Nursing.* Philadelphia, Pa: WB Saunders Co; 1998:566–579.

97. Carpenito-Moyet L-J. *Nursing Diagnosis: Application to Clinical Practice.* 10th ed. Philadelphia, Pa: Lippincott; 2004.

98. Welch WC, Jacobs GB. Surgery for metastatic spinal disease. *J Neurol Oncol* 1995;23:163–170.

99. Schulam PG, Kawashima A, Sandler C, et al. Urinary tract imaging: basic principles. In: Walsh PC, Retik AS, Vaughan ED Jr, eds. *Campbell's Urology.* 8th ed. Philadelphia, Pa: WB Saunders; 2002:122–166.

100. Sullano MA, Ortiz EJ. Deep vein thrombosis and anticoagulant therapy. *Nurs Clin North Am.* 2001;36:645–663.

101. Nakashima J, Tachibana M, Veno M, et al. Tumor necrosis factor and coagulopathy in patients with prostate cancer. *Cancer Res.* 1995;55:8881–8885.

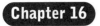

The Use of Complementary and Alternative Therapies in Men with Prostate Cancer

INTRODUCTION[1-6]

Definition of Complementary and Alternative (CAM)
- Multiple, varied, and diverse
- The intent with which it is used is what defines a CAM therapy
  - A therapy is considered *complementary* when it is used to complement conventional medicine.
  - A therapy is considered *alternative* when it is used instead of conventional medicine.
  - Integrative or integrated therapy is a contemporary term for the use of a complementary therapy or therapies with conventional medicine.

Uses[7]
- Reduce therapy-related side effects
- Improve patient tolerance to cancer therapy
- Enhance quality of life

CAM Use[8-9]
- Approximately 27–39% of prostate cancer patients use CAM therapies

CAM Categories
- See **Table 16–1**.
- Some CAM therapies are in clinical trials.[10]

CAM AND EVIDENCE–BASED PRACTICE
- The amount of evidence-based practice related to CAM therapies is limited but is increasing.
- Data on efficacy and safety are also limited for some.
- The number of patients using CAM therapies is increasing due to its ready availability.
- Making CAM therapy suggestions is complicated by the limited amount of data and supporting evidence related to efficacy and safety.
- Patients may obtain CAM information from a wide variety of very unreliable resources.
- See **Figure 16–1** for an algorithm to use when discussing CAM therapies with patients.
- Patients with prostate cancer that were found to be interested in CAM therapies[11]
  - Minority ethnic group
  - Higher education

And the patients did not share information related to CAM usage with their physician.

Table 16–1 NCI OCCAM Domains of CAM and Modalities in Clinical Trials

Domain	Definition
Alternative medical systems	Systems built upon complete systems of theory and practice
Manipulative and body-based methods	Methods based on manipulation and/or movement of one or more parts of the body
Energy therapies	Therapies involving the use of energy fields
Mind-body interventions	Techniques designed to enhance the mind's capacity to affect bodily function and symptoms
Movement therapy	Modalities used to improve patterns of bodily movement
Nutritional therapeutics	Assortment of nutrients and nonnutrient and bioactive food components that are used as chemopreventative agents, and the use of specific foods or diets as cancer prevention or treatment strategies
Pharmacological and biological treatments	Drugs, complex natural products, vaccines, and other biological interventions not yet accepted in mainstream medicine; off-label use of prescription drugs
Complex natural products	Subcategory of pharmacological and biological treatments consisting of an assortment of plant samples (botanicals), extracts of crude natural substances, and unfractionate extracts from marine organisms used for healing and treatment of disease

Data compiled from Decker and Lee[7]; PDQ.[10]

Example(s)	Modality in Clinical Trials	
Traditional Chinese medicine (acupuncture), Ayurveda, homeopathy, naturopathy, Tibetan medicine	• Acupuncture • Electroacupuncture	• Acupressure • Traumeel S
Chiropractic, therapeutic massage, osteopathy, reflexology	• Distance healing • Group therapy • Music therapy • Standard counseling	• Exercise-based counseling • Healing touch • Spirituality, religiosity • Stress management training
Reiki, Therapeutic Touch, pulsed fields, magnet therapy	• Energy healing • Reiki	• Energy therapy • Touch
Meditation, hypnosis, art therapy, biofeedback, mental healing, imagery, relaxation therapy, support groups, music therapy, cognitive-behavioral therapy, prayer, dance therapy, psychoneuroimmunology, aromatherapy, animal-assisted therapy	Distance healing, exercise-based counseling, group therapy, healing touch, music therapy, spirituality, and religiosity	
T'ai chi, Feldenkrais, Hatha yoga, Alexander technique, dance therapy, qigong, rolfing, Trager method, applied kinesiology	None	
Dietary regimens such as macrobiotics, vegetarian, Gerson therapy, Kelley/Gonzalez regimen, vitamins, dietary macronutrients, supplements, antioxidants, melatonin, selenium, coenzyme Q10, ephedra, ortho-molecular medicine	• Black cohosh • Curcumin • Folic acid • Garlic • Herbal therapy • L-carnitine • Lycopene • Noni fruit extract • Pomegranate juice • Soy protein isolate • Vitamins C and E	• Creatine • Flax seed • Fruit and vegetable extracts • Ginger • Juven • Low-fat diet • Macrobiotic diet • Nutritional supplements • Selenium • Valeriana *officinalis* • Zinc sulfate
Antineoplastons, products from honey bees, 714-X, low-dose naltrexone, metenkephalin, immunoaugmentative therapy, laetrile, hydrazine sulfate, New Castle virus, melatonin, ozone therapy, thymus therapy, enzyme therapy, high-dose vitamin C	Antineoplastons Pancreatic proteolytic enzymes	
Herbs and herbal extracts, mixtures of tea polyphenols, shark cartilage, Essiac tea, cordyceps, Sun Soup, MGN-3	• Chinese herbal extract • Kanglaite injection • Mistletoe • Shark cartilage • Virulizin	• Green tea extract (polyphenon E) • Milk thistle • Pycnogenol • St. John's wort

Source: Decker GM. The use of complementary and alternative (CAM) therapies in men with prostate cancer. In: Held-Warmkessel, J., ed. *Contemporary Issues in Prostate Cancer: A Nursing Perspective* (2nd ed). Jones and Bartlett Publishers, 2006, 392–415. Reprinted with permission by Jones and Bartlett Publishers.

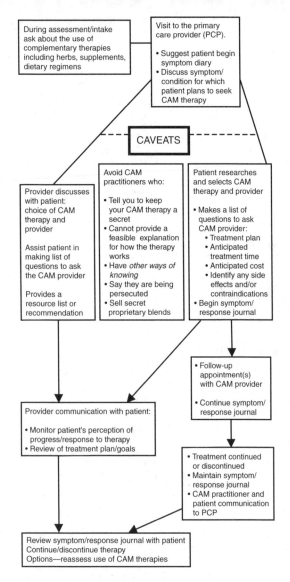

Figure 16-1. Algorithm discussing CAM therapies with patients
Source: Decker G. Integrating complementary and alternative medicine therapies into an ambulatory practice. In: Buchsel P, Yarbro CH, eds. *Oncology Nursing in the Ambulatory Setting.* Sudbury, MA: Jones and Bartlett Publishers; 2004:355–376. Reprinted with permission by Jones and Bartlett Publishers.

THE OLDER ADULT WITH CANCER[12-15]

- Patient variables that may influence use of CAM therapies
  - Age
  - Education
  - Stage of disease
  - Religion
  - Ethnic group
  - Culture
  - Financial resources
  - Family, friends, and third-party payors
- Including CAM therapies may complicate the patients' decision-making processes regarding conventional cancer therapy.
- Information-seeking behaviors of older adults and where they obtain the information may influence their decision making. Patients need reliable sources of information, and their health care provider may not have sufficient knowledge on the CAM therapies the patient is considering. See **Table 16–2** for reliable Web site resources.
- CAM may be considered by patients for initial cancer therapy, at time of disease relapse, or for symptom management. (See **Table 16–3**. [16-59])

Comorbidities

- Comorbidities must be considered with decision making when considering use of CAM therapies.
- Drug-drug, drug-herb, drug-vitamin, and herb-vitamin interactions must be evaluated.
  - Many interactions remain undetermined.
- Nurses must encourage patients to fully disclose all CAM therapy use.
- CAM therapies may have known and unknown interactions with conventional cancer therapies.

Confusion About CAM Therapies

- Confusions surrounding CAM therapies may be based on false assumptions made by patients about CAM therapies.
  - Patients may assume that because a herb is a natural product that it is therefore safe for them to use.
  - Patients may assume that a CAM therapy is specific to a diagnosis or symptom.
- Some CAM therapies may be safe to use with certain types of cancer therapies, and others may not be safe to use with any cancer therapies.

Contraindications and Warnings About Use with Conventional Therapies

- Antioxidants are thought to interfere with a number of cancer therapies, including (but not limited to) radiation therapy, alkylating agents, antimetabolites, and taxanes, and must be avoided.
- Certain herbs may interfere with the efficacy of a number of chemotherapy agents and biotherapy agents, and must be avoided (see **Table 16–4**[60-89]).
- The length of time certain CAM therapies must be avoided is not known for many conventional cancer therapies. Patients need to be encouraged to disclose CAM use with all their health care providers.
- Patients on phase I studies must not take any other products, treatments, herbs, supplements, or medications without the approval of the treating physician.

TABLE 16–2 Examples of Selected Sources for Reliable Cancer CAM Information

Sponsored Web Sites	
American Cancer Society	http://www.cancer.org
American Society for Clinical Oncology	http://www.asco.org
National Institutes of Health	http://www.nih.gov
* Cancer Information Service	http://cis.nci.nih.gov
* Office of Cancer Complementary and Alternative Medicine	http://www3.cancer.gov/occam
* National Center for Complementary and Alternative Medicine	http://nccam.nih.gov
* Office of Dietary Supplements	http://ods.od.nih.gov
* Medline Plus	http://medlineplus.gov
* Cancer Patient Education Network	http://cpen.nci.nih.gov
* People Living with Cancer	http://www.plwc.org
Selected Sponsored Databases	
Complementary and Alternative Medicine and Pain Database	http://www.campain.umm.edu/News.html
Food & Drug Administration	http://www.fda.gov
Herbalgram.org	http://www.herbalgram.org/
International Bibliographic Information on Dietary Supplements	http://dietary-supplements.info.nih.gov/databases/ibids.html
Natural Medicine	http://www.naturaldatabase.com/
Natural Standard	http://www.naturalstandard.com/
PDQ	http://cancer.gov/cancerinfo/pdq/
The Cochrane Collaboration	http://www.cochrane.org/index0.htm

Adapted from Decker and Lee.[7]
Source: Decker GM. The use of complementary and alternative (CAM) therapies in men with prostate cancer. In: Held-Warmkessel, J., ed. *Contemporary Issues in Prostate Cancer: A Nursing Perspective* (2nd ed). Jones and Bartlett Publishers, 2006, 392–415. Reprinted with permission by Jones and Bartlett Publishers.

Safety and Liability

- Patients may use CAM therapies to treat comorbidities and fail to disclose their CAM use thinking that its use may not be important to their cancer care.
- Patients may use specific CAM therapies to treat prostate cancer (see **Table 16–4**).
- Liability is a concern and consideration for nurses who recommend a CAM therapy provider who may not have appropriate credentials.[90–91]

TABLE 16–3 Examples of Common Symptom Management Considerations in Cancer CAM

Traditional Approach(es) and Outcome(s)	CAM Approach(es) and Outcome(s)
Antidepressants/depression Tricyclic antidepressants and selective serotonin reuptake inhibitors (SSRIs) demonstrate efficacy in the treatment of depression	**Acupuncture** *seems to decrease symptoms of depression* Three RCTs demonstrated efficacy of eletroacupuncture as similar to tricyclic antidepressants.[16,17] RCTs using nonspecific (sham) acupuncture show conflicting results.[18] Acupuncture improved the course of depression more than pharmacological treatment with mianserin alone in an RCT of 70 inpatients with a major depressive episode in three different treatment groups: verum acupuncture, placebo acupuncture, and a control group. All three groups were pharmacologically treated with the antidepressant mianserin.[19]
Counseling psychotherapy Counseling and psychotherapy are common effective interventions for depression	*Surveys have identified depression as one of the most common reasons for using CAM. The most popular therapies are exercise, herbal medicine, relaxation, and spiritual healing.*[20,21] **Herbal therapies** St. John's wort (SJW) is effective in the treatment of mild to moderate depression.[18,22–24] The value of SJW in severe depression is questionable.[24] There are multiple actual and potential drug–herb interactions and contraindications. Should not be used with chemotherapy or biotherapy without physician approval and knowledge.
Physical therapy when appropriate	**Autogenic training** When utilized as a single therapy (2/week x 10 weeks) resulted in reduction in symptoms similar to psychotherapy alone but not significantly more than with no intervention. Authors warned that autogenic training alone is not recommended as treatment for depression.[25]
Music therapy Patients with cancer are among those who can benefit from music as a therapy. Music provides unique opportunities and properties that promote well-being. Music has been effective in the treatment of the anxiety and fear associated with a cancer diagnosis and cancer therapy.[26–29] Psychoneuroimmunology identifies potential implications for cancer care.[30–32]	**Music therapy** Patients with cancer are among those who can benefit from music as a therapy. Music provides unique opportunities and properties that promote well-being. Music has been effective in the treatment of the anxiety and fear associated with a cancer diagnosis and cancer therapy.[26–29] Psychoneuroimmunology identifies potential implications for cancer care.[30–32]

continues

TABLE 16–3 Examples of Common Symptom Management Considerations in Cancer CAM, continued

Traditional Approach(es) and Outcome(s)	CAM Approach(es) and Outcome(s)
Massage Massage (qd x 5 days) was more effective than viewing videos in children and adolescents. Improvements were measured symptoms of depression, anxiety, sleep, and cortisol levels.[33] Massage should be used with caution when a patient has a history of abuse, PTSD, and other psychiatric disorders.[34–36]	**Massage** Massage (qd x 5 days) was more effective than viewing videos in children and adolescents. Improvements were measured symptoms of depression, anxiety, sleep, and cortisol levels.[33] Massage should be used with caution when a patient has a history of abuse, PTSD, and other psychiatric disorders.[34–36]
	Exercise There is a large body of research, considered to be of questionable quality that support the antidepressant effects of exercise. There are RCTs that provide verification of the efficacy of exercise in the treatment of depression. Aerobic and nonaerobic forms of exercise have proven to be effective. In three RCTs data suggest that aerobic exercise may be as effective as psychological or drug treatment. The exact mechanisms are not known.[37]
	Dance and movement therapy Dance and movement therapy are effective therapeutic interventions in reducing symptoms of depression and improving psychological well-being.[38–42]
Surgery Curative excision or palliative debulking can relieve symptoms of obstruction or compression, improve prognosis, and may increase survival.[43]	**Acupuncture** National Institutes of Health Acupuncture Consensus Development Panel concluded that acupuncture may be useful for headache and low-back pain.[44]
Antineoplastic therapy Antineoplastic therapy (chemotherapy, biological, or hormonal therapy) may provide palliation by reducing tumor burden.[45] Chemotherapy is effective in prolonging time to disease progression and survival in patients with advanced colorectal cancer.[46]	**Cognitive–Behavioral Treatment (CBT)** Standard CBT (five 50-minute sessions) and profile-tailored CBT (based on results from biobehavioral pain profile [measures factors related to pain experience]) showed greater improvement in pain relief than usual care.[47]
Radiation therapy Local or whole-body radiation enhances the effectiveness of analgesics and noninvasive therapies to relieve cancer pain. Single injections of beta particle-emitting agents can relieve pain secondary to bony metastases.[43]	**Chiropractic** SR of chiropractic manipulation for back, neck, headache disorders, nonspinal pain syndromes (excluding headache) failed to demonstrated efficacy.[48]
Nonsteroidal anti-inflammatory drugs (NSAIDs) NSAIDs appear to be more effective than placebo for cancer pain. Combinations of an NSAID with an opioid have shown either no or slight significant difference compared with either single intervention.[49]	**Massage** RCTs using Swedish massage suggest efficacy for relieving back pain; however, the results were not uniform.[48]

TABLE 16–3 Examples of Common Symptom Management Considerations in Cancer CAM, continued

Traditional Approach(es) and Outcome(s)	CAM Approach(es) and Outcome(s)
Opioids Uncontrolled case series show that chronic pain (not associated with terminal disease) is relieved by a stable nonescalating dose of opioids with minimal risk of addiction. Opioids can induce abnormal pain sensitivity. Prolonged high-dose opioid therapy may have serious adverse sequelae (tolerance, sensitivity, hormonal effects, immunosuppression). Remaining questions: are opioids beneficial over years (versus months) and does the dose of the opioid have an effect on the efficacy and safety of long-term therapy?[50]	**Relaxation with guided imagery** Relaxation with guided imagery can improve oral mucositis.[51] Relaxation exercises are effective: slow rhythmic breathing; touch and massage; reflecting on peaceful past experiences; listening to music.[43]
Transcutaneous electrical nerve stimulation (TENS) TENS may be effective for the treatment of neuropathic pain.[52]	**Topical capsaicin** Moderate to poor efficacy in the treatment of chronic musculoskeletal or neuropathic pain. May be useful as an adjunct or sole therapy for pain that is unresponsive to other treatments.[53]
Antidepressants SR of antidepressants suggest efficacy in the treatment of neuropathic pain over placebo. First choice of drug class of antidepressants is uncertain.[54]	**Physical modalities** Musculoskeletal pain may be treated with heat, cold, massage, and exercise therapy.[43]
Neurolytic blocks Effective in controlling cancer pain in select patients in addition to pharmacological therapy. Quality improves when placement is image-guided in collaboration with an interventional radiologist.[55]	**Music versus distraction** Lack of definitive findings in RCT using music or distraction for controlling procedural pain versus standard approach (neither music or distraction).[28]
Topical rubefacients containing salicylates Moderate to poor efficacy in the treatment of musculoskeletal and arthritic pain.[56]	**Percutaneous electrical nerve stimulation (PENS)** PENS (acupuncture-like needle probes plus nerve stimulation) can be a useful supplement to opioids in the management of bony metastases and pain.[57]
Biphosphonates Biphosphonates have a role in managing refractory pain from metastases where oncologic or orthopedic intervention is delayed or inappropriate.[58]	**Distraction** Distraction via paced auditory serial addition task (mental math) was shown to inhibit pain perception.[59]
Distraction Distraction via paced auditory serial addition task (mental math) was shown to inhibit pain perception.[59]	

RCT, randomized clinical trial; PTSD, post-traumatic stress disorder.
Adapted from Decker and Lee.[7]

Source: Decker GM. The use of complementary and alternative (CAM) therapies in men with prostate cancer. In: Held-Warmkessel, J., ed. *Contemporary Issues in Prostate Cancer: A Nursing Perspective* (2nd ed). Jones and Bartlett Publishers, 2006, 392–415. Reprinted with permission by Jones and Bartlett Publishers.

TABLE 16–4 Examples of CAM Therapies Used in the Treatment and/or Management of Prostate Cancer

Therapy/Description	Indications/Contraindications/Level of Evidence
Herbals	
Camelia senesis (green tea)	In a recently reported case-control study conducted in China, the prostate cancer risk was shown to decline with increasing frequency, duration, and quantity of green tea consumption. The researchers reported that the dose–response relationships were also significant, suggesting that green tea is protective against prostate cancer.[60]
	Decaffeinated green tea (DGT) is unlikely to alter the disposition of medications primarily dependent on the CYP2D6 or CYP3A4 pathways of metabolism.[61]
	Benefits of specific doses of green tea are not established. Most studies have examined green tea in the form of a brewed beverage, rather than in capsule form.
	Some research suggests cancer-protective properties of habitual green tea consumption, while others have not observed significant benefits. Animal and laboratory research suggests that components of green tea may actually be carcinogenic[62] (although not specific to prostate cancer). However, at this time, the scientific evidence remains undetermined.[61]
	Direction of evidence: inconclusive
	Level of risk: Studies of the side effects of green tea are limited. However, green tea contains caffeine, for which reactions have been reported.[61]
	Contraindication: In those with known allergy/hypersensitivity to caffeine or tannin, green tea should be avoided. Skin rash and hives have been reported with caffeine ingestion.[61]
PC-SPES (PC = prostate cancer/ SPES = hope); composed of 8 herbs	Estrogenic effects were demonstrated *in vitro*,[63] in mice[63, 64] and in humans.[63, 65] *In vitro* studies have demonstrated that it inhibits growth of various cell-lines including androgen-sensitive and androgen-insensitive prostate cancer cells.[60]
	Studies showed a decrease in prostate-specific antigen (PSA) levels,[64] stabilized or decreased metastases,[66] reduced pain,[67] and improved quality of life.[67]
	Reported adverse effects have been contributed to estrogenic effects.[64, 65, 67–69] Reports of product contamination with conventional medications[63, 70] caused the results to be questioned. That is, were the results obtained due to the herbal combination or a contaminant such as DES or warfarin.[63, 69]
	No data available on use with chemotherapy or radiation therapy.[69]
	Direction of evidence: Preliminary evidence was positive; however, use was associated with major adverse events. Recalled by manufacturer. No longer available.[69]

TABLE 16–4 Examples of CAM Therapies Used in the Treatment and/or Management of Prostate Cancer, continued

Therapy/Description	Indications/Contraindications/Level of Evidence
Rasagenthi lehyam (RL) Contains 38 botanicals, 8 inorganic compounds, palm sugar,[16] and hen's egg base.[20]	Preliminary data validated anticancer activity (*in vitro*) of RL when used as an alternative prostate cancer therapy, as a radiation sensitizer, and as a complementary medicine in the treatment of prostate cancer.[20]
	Direction of evidence: Positive but inconclusive[20] from one RCT.[20]
	Level of risk: Not yet determined[20]
Diet supplements	
Vitamin E	For latent prostate cancer
	Direction of evidence: Positive[69] from more than one (properly designed) RCT [69, 71]
	Level of risk: Low (theoretical risk of adverse event is low)[69]
	Contraindications: Avoid concurrent use with radiation therapy and certain chemotherapy.[69] (Those believed to have a higher theoretical risk are those that rely on free radicals and reactive oxygen species.[69, 72, 73])
	For other than latent prostate cancer
	It is considered plausible that vitamin E may help in primary cancer prevention.[69, 74] Mechanisms/role in cancer progression not known.[69]
Other antioxidants	It is believed that antioxidants can help in primary cancer prevention because oxidative cell damage might increase the risk for cancer.[75] This includes vitamin A (and all precursors) and vitamin C as well as vitamin E. Their role in cancer progression is not clear.[69]
	Direction of evidence: Inconclusive. Based on the opinions of respected authorities +/− descriptive studies[69, 72]
	Level of risk is low.[69]
	Contraindications: Avoid concurrent use with radiation therapy, certain chemotherapy.[69] (Those believed to have a higher theoretical risk are those that rely on free radicals and reactive oxygen species.[69, 72, 73])
Saw palmetto	Saw palmetto (*Serenoa repens, Sabal serrulata*) is used popularly in Europe for symptoms associated with benign prostatic hypertrophy (enlargement of the prostate). Although not considered standard of care in the United States, it is the most popular herbal treatment for this condition.
	Multiple mechanisms of action have been proposed, and saw palmetto appears to possess 5-α-reductase inhibitory activity (thereby preventing the conversion of testosterone to dihydrotestosterone).

continues

TABLE 16–4 Examples of CAM Therapies Used in the Treatment and/or Management of Prostate Cancer, continued

Therapy/Description	Indications/Contraindications/Level of Evidence
Saw palmetto, cont'd	Hormonal/estrogenic effects have also been reported, as well as direct inhibitory effects on androgen receptors and anti-inflammatory properties.
	Saw palmetto has not been thoroughly compared to other types of drugs used for benign prostatic hypertrophy (BPH). Most available studies have assessed the standardized saw palmetto product Permixon.[61]
	Overall, the available scientific evidence favors the effectiveness of saw palmetto for BPH and not for prostate cancer even though it was one of the ingredients in PC-SPES.[61]
	There have been reports describing men with prostate cancer who developed deep vein thromboses and pulmonary emboli while taking saw palmetto. It has not been determined if saw palmetto was the cause.[61]
	Direction of evidence: Positive for BPH, not for prostate cancer.
	Level of risk: Saw palmetto can cause a false negative or decrease in PSA levels.
	Few incidents of severe side effects of saw palmetto are noted in the published scientific literature. The most common include stomach pain, nausea, vomiting, bad breath, constipation, or diarrhea.[61, 74]
Selenium	Follow-up results of the Nutritional Prevention of Cancer Trial (NPC) have recently been prereleased online ahead of paper publication in the *British Journal of Cancer* (June 22, 2004).
	A growing body of literature suggests that selenium supplementation reduces the risk of developing prostate cancer in men with normal baseline PSA (prostate-specific antigen) levels, and low blood selenium levels. This is the subject of large well-designed studies, including the Nutritional Prevention of Cancer Trial (NPC), and the ongoing Selenium and Vitamin E Cancer Prevention Trial (SELECT), as well as prior population and case-control studies.
	The complete (13 year) results of the Nutritional Prevention of Cancer Trial have been analyzed,[76] causing some speculation over the robustness of the previously reported findings of reduction of cancer risks by supplements of selenium (Se) to a cohort of older Americans. These analysis confirmed that Se supplementation was associated with marked reductions in risks to total (all sites except skin) carcinomas and to cancers of

TABLE 16-4 Examples of CAM Therapies Used in the Treatment and/or Management of Prostate Cancer, continued

Therapy/Description	Indications/Contraindications/Level of Evidence
Selenium, cont'd	the prostate and colon-rectum. Of those deep-site treatment effects, the most robust was for prostate cancer, which was more frequent, and was confirmed by serum prostate-specific antigen level. Recent subgroup analyses showed Se supplementation reduced risk of cancer mostly among subjects who entered the trial with plasma Se levels in the bottom tertile of the cohort. Other recent findings have demonstrated that Se treatment can promote apoptosis in prostate cancer cells and, possibly, impair their proliferation through antiangiogenic effects. Thus, a body of basic understanding is developing by which one can understand and evaluate the results of the Nutritional Prevention of Cancer and future clinical trials. This understanding also requires inclusion of the mechanisms of Se transport and cellular uptake so that appropriate inferences can be made from findings from cell culture systems, which tended to use effective Se doses much larger than relevant to cells *in vivo*. Also needed is information on the chemical speciation of Se in foods, so that Se delivery can be achieved in ways that are effective in reducing cancer risk and is also safe, accessible, and sustainable.[61, 76] Direction of evidence: Positive Level of risk: Low Caution regarding doses that exceed the recommended 200–400 mcg/day[74]
Shark cartilage	Patients with cancer use shark cartilage products that are administered orally or rectally. It is believed that since the active ingredients are proteins or glycoproteins it would be difficult for these substances to enter the circulatory system. There is one report of the presence of proteins after oral administration.[77] Shark cartilage has antiangiogenesis properties.[69, 21] Current clinical evidence does not support the use of this substance in the treatment of cancer.[69] Direction of evidence: Inconclusive Level of risk: Low, unless patient has hypercalcemia or when antiangiogenesis might be detrimental.[69, 78] Common side effects are gastrointestinal symptoms.[78] Generally well tolerated. No interaction with radiation therapy or chemotherapy known.[69]

continues

TABLE 16–4 Examples of CAM Therapies Used in the Treatment and/or Management of Prostate Cancer, continued

Therapy/Description	Indications/Contraindications/Level of Evidence
Soy—a major dietary source of isoflavonoid phytoestrogens	Believed to contribute to protective effects on progression of latent prostate cancer.[69]
	Mechanisms include weak estrogenic effects, may limit impact of endogenous sex hormones, compete with estradiol for binding sites. Inhibits enzymes needed for androgen synthesis (decreasing activity of androgens).[79–80] It is unclear if this would occur at significant concentrations in humans.[81]
	RCTs do not support the reduction of testosterone by isoflavinoid action on hypothalamus and pituitary gland.[79, 81]
	The pro-estrogenic effects might provide benefits in prostate cancer. There are no published studies that evaluate the effect of soy on prostate cancer progression.[69]
	Because isoflavonoids have antioxidant activity, combining them with radiation and/or chemotherapy is not recommended.[82] Avoid in those patients who are thrombocytopenic, have clotting disorders, or taking anticoagulants. Isoflavones have been shown to have antiplatelet activity in primates.[69, 83]
	Direction of evidence: Inconclusive, based on the opinions of respected authorities[69]
	Level of risk: Low[69, 80]
Isoflavone genistein	Potential antitumor effects extend beyond sex hormone interactions, including, inhibition of tyrosine kinases,[84] suppression of cell proliferation *in vitro*,[80, 85] and *in vitro* inhibition of angiogenesis[85]
	There are mixed results in animal studies of oral genistein supplementation in hormone dependent cancers.[69, 86]
	Direction of evidence: inconclusive[69]
	Level of risk: Low[69]
Diet	
Reduced dietary fat intake	Studies have shown a relationship between the American diet and the progression of a latent prostate cancer to the clinical stage.[87] Specifically, there is a definite association between saturated or animal fat and the progression of prostate cancer.[69, 88, 89]

Source: Decker GM. The use of complementary and alternative (CAM) therapies in men with prostate cancer. In: Held-Warmkessel, J., ed. *Contemporary Issues in Prostate Cancer: A Nursing Perspective* (2nd ed). Jones and Bartlett Publishers, 2006, 392–415. Reprinted with permission by Jones and Bartlett Publishers.

I thank Georgia Decker, MS, RN, CS-ANP, CN, AOCN, for her review of this chapter.

References

1. Vickers AJ, Cassileth BR. Unconventional therapies for cancer and cancer-related symptoms. *Lancet Oncol.* 2001;2:226–232.
2. Cassileth BR, Vickers AJ. Complementary and alternative therapies. *Urol Clin North Am.* 2003;30:369–376.
3. Ernst E. Complementary therapies for cancer. Available at: http://www.uptodateonline .com/application/topic/print.asp?file=genl_onc/8402. Accessed April 12, 2004.
4. NCCAM. National Center for Complementary and Alternative Medicine. Available at: http://nccam.nih.gov/. Accessed May 8, 2004.
5. Cassileth BR. 'Complementary' or 'alternative'? It makes a difference in cancer care. *Complement Ther Med.* 1999;7:35–37.
6. Oncology Nursing Society. *The Use of Complementary and Alternative Therapies in Cancer Care.* Pittsburgh, Pa: Oncology Nursing Society; 2002.
7. Decker GL, Lee CO. Complementary and alternative medicine (CAM) therapies. In: Yarbro CH, Goodman M, Frogge M, eds. *Cancer Nursing: Principles and Practice.* 6th ed. Sudbury, Mass: Jones and Bartlett; 2005:590–615.
8. Boon H, Brown JB, Gavin A, et al. Men with prostate cancer: making decisions about complementary / alternative medicine. *Medical Decision Making.* 2003 (Nov–Dec):471–479.
9. Nam RK, Fleshner N, Rakovitch E, et al. Prevalence and patterns of the use of complementary therapies among prostate cancer patients: an epidemiological analysis. *J Urol.* 1999;161:1521–1524.
10. PDQ. PDQ Cancer Information Summaries: Complementary and Alternative Medicine. Available at: http://www.cancer.gov/cancerinfo/pdq/cam. Accessed April 13, 2004.
11. Diefenbach MA, Hamerick N, Uzzo R, et al. Clinical, demographic, and psychosocial correlates of complementary and alternative medicine use by men diagnosed with localized prostate cancer. *J Urol.* 2003;170:166–169.
12. Schulz R, Heckhausen J. A lifespan model of successful aging. *Am J Psychol.* 1996;51:702–708.
13. Llewelyn-Thomas HA, McGrew J, et al. Cancer patients' decision making and trial entry preferences: the effects of framing information about short-term toxicity and long-term survival. *Med Decision Making.* 1995;15:836–847.
14. Polsky D, Keating NL, Weeks JC, et al. Patient choice of breast cancer treatment: impact on health state preferences. *Modern Care.* 2002;40:1068–1079.
15. Goodman M. Patient's view count as well. *Nursing Standard.* 1995;9:40–55.
16. Luo HC, Jia YK, Li Z. Electro-acupuncture vs. amitriptyline in the treatment of depressive states. *J Tradit Chin Med.* 1985;5:3–8.
17. Lynch EP, Lazor MA, Gellis JE, et al. The impact of postoperative pain on the development of postoperative delirium. *Anesth Analg.* 1998;86:781–785.
18. Ernst E (ed.) *The Desktop Guide to Complementary and Alternative Medicine: An Evidence-Based Approach.* Edinburgh, UK: Mosby; 2001.
19. Roschke J, Wolf C, Muller MJ, et al. The benefit from whole body acupuncture in major depression. *J Affect Disord.* 2000;57:73–81.
20. Ranga RS, Ramankuttym G, Nur-e-alan M, et al. A novel complementary and alternative medicine for prostate cancer. *Cancer Chemothero Pharmacol.* 2004;54:7–15.
21. Herbal P. *PDR for Herbal Medicines.* Montvale, NJ: Medical Economics Company; 2001.

22. Stevinson C. Why patients use complementary and alternative medicine. In: Ernst E, ed. *The Desktop Guide to Complementary and Alternative Medicine: An Evidence-Based Approach*. Edinburg, UK: Harcourt Publishers Limited; 2001.

23. Kasper S, Dienel A. Cluster analysis of symptoms during antidepressant treatment with Hypericum extract in mildly to moderately depressed out-patients. A meta-analysis of data from three randomized, placebo-controlled trials. *Psychopharmacology (Berl)*. 2002;164:301–308.

24. Whiskey E, Werneke U, Taylor D. A systematic review and meta-analysis of Hypericum perforatum in depression: a comprehensive clinical review. *Int Clin Psychopharmacol*. 2001;16:239–252.

25. Krampen G, Main C, Waelbroeck O. [Optimizing the learning process in short-term autogenic training by practice protocols]. *Z Klin Psychol Psychopathol Psychother*. 1991;39:33–45.

26. Burns DS. The effect of the bonny method of guided imagery and music on the mood and life quality of cancer patients. *J Music Ther*. 2001;38:51–65.

27. Cassileth BR, Vickers AJ, Magill LA. Music therapy for mood disturbance during hospitalization for autologous stem cell transplantation: a randomized controlled trial. *Cancer*. 2003;98:2723–2729.

28. Beck SL. The therapeutic use of music for cancer-related pain. *Oncol Nurs Forum*. 1991;18:1327–1337.

29. Kwekkeboom KL. Music versus distraction for procedural pain and anxiety in patients with cancer. *Oncol Nurs Forum*. 2003;30:433–440.

30. Zappa SB, Cassileth BR. Complementary approaches to palliative oncological care. *J Nurs Care Qual*. 2003;18:22–26.

31. Hilliard RE. The effects of music therapy on the quality and length of life of people diagnosed with terminal cancer. *J Music Ther*. 2003;40:113–137.

32. Yamashita A, Kato S. [Music therapy used on a patient in the terminal stage of cancer who narrated a tale based on her fantasy]. *Seishin Shinkeigaku Zasshi*. 2003;105:787–794.

33. Platania-Solazzo A, Field TM, Blank J, et al. Relaxation therapy reduces anxiety in child and adolescent psychiatric patients. *Acta Paedopsychiatr*. 1992;55:115–120.

34. Moyer CA, Rounds J, Hannum JW. A meta-analysis of massage therapy research. *Psychol Bull*. 2004;130:3–18.

35. Jorm AF, Christensen H, Griffiths KM, et al. Effectiveness of complementary and self-help treatments for depression. *Med J Aust*. 2002;176(suppl):S84–S96.

36. Rexilius SJ, Mundt C, Erickson Megel M, et al. Therapeutic effects of massage therapy and handling touch on caregivers of patients undergoing autologous hematopoietic stem cell transplant. *Oncol Nurs Forum*. 2002;29:E35–E44.

37. Crevenna R, Zielinski C, Keilani MY, et al. [Aerobic endurance training for cancer patients]. *Wien Med Wochenschr*. 2003;153:212–216.

38. Ernst E, Rand JI, Stevinson C. Complementary therapies for depression: an overview. *Arch Gen Psychiatry*. 1998;55:1026–1032.

39. Estivill M. Therapeutic aspects of aerobic dance participation. *Health Care Women Int*. 1995;16:341–350.

40. Ostwald PF, Baron BC, Byl NM, et al. Performing arts medicine. *West J Med*. 1994;160:48–52.

41. Pappas GP, Golin S, Meyer DL. Reducing symptoms of depression with exercise. *Psychosomatics*. 1990;31:112–113.

42 Gurley V, Neuringer A, Massee J. Dance and sports compared: effects on psychological well-being. *J Sports Med Phys Fitness.* 1984;24:58–68.

43. NCI. Pain. *National Cancer Institute.* Available at: http://www.nci.nih.gov/cancerinfo/pdq/supportivecare. Accessed May 18, 2004.

44. Mayer DJ. Acupuncture: an evidence-based review of the clinical literature. *Annu Rev Med.* 2000;51:49–63.

45. Paice JA. Pain. In: Yarbro CH, Frogge MH, Goodman M, eds. *Cancer Symptom Management.* Sudbury, Mass: Jones and Bartlett Publishers; 2004.

46. Simmonds PC. Palliative chemotherapy for advanced colorectal cancer: systematic review and meta-analysis. Colorectal Cancer Collaborative Group. *BMJ.* 2000;321:531–535.

47. Dalton JA, Keefe FJ, Carlson J, et al. Tailoring cognitive-behavioral treatment for cancer pain. *Pain Manag Nurs.* 2004;5:3–18.

48. Ernst E. Manual therapies for pain control: chiropractic and massage. *Clin J Pain.* 2004;20:8–12.

49. McNicol E, Strassels S, Goudas L, et al. Nonsteroidal anti-inflammatory drugs, alone or combined with opioids, for cancer pain: a systematic review *J Clin Oncol.* 2004;22:1975–1992.

50. Ballantyne JC, Mao J. Opioid therapy for chronic pain. *N Engl J Med.* 2003;349:1943–1953.

51. Pan CX, Morrison RS, Ness J, et al. Complementary and alternative medicine in the management of pain, dyspnea, and nausea and vomiting near the end of life. A systematic review. *J Pain Symptom Manage.* 2000;20:374–387.

52. Martin LA, Hagen NA. Neuropathic pain in cancer patients: mechanisms, syndromes, and clinical controversies. *J Pain Symptom Manage.* 1997;14:99–117.

53. Mason L, Moore RA, Derry S, et al. Systematic review of topical capsaicin for the treatment of chronic pain. *BMJ.* 2004;328:991. Epub 2004 Mar 219.

54. McQuay HJ, Tramer M, Nye BA, Carroll D, Wiffen PJ, Moore RA. A systematic review of antidepressants in neuropathic pain. *Pain.* 1996;68:217–227.

55. Kongsgaard UE, Bjorgo S, Hauser M. [Neurolytic blocks for cancer pain—still a useful therapeutic strategy]. *Tidsskr Nor Laegeforen.* 2004;124:481–483.

56. Mason L, Moore RA, Edwards JE, et al. Systematic review of efficacy of topical rubefacients containing salicylates for the treatment of acute and chronic pain. *BMJ.* 2004;328:995. Epub 2004 Mar 219.

57. Ahmed HE, Craig WF, White PF, et al. Percutaneous electrical nerve stimulation (PENS): a complementary therapy for the management of pain secondary to bony metastasis. *Clin J Pain.* 1998;14:320–323.

58. Mannix K, Ahmedzai SH, Anderson H, et al. Using bisphosphonates to control the pain of bone metastases: evidence-based guidelines for palliative care. *Palliat Med.* 2000;14:455–461.

59. Terkelsen AJ, Andersen OK, Molgaard H, et al. Mental stress inhibits pain perception and heart rate variability but not a nociceptive withdrawal reflex. *Acta Physiol Scand.* 2004;180:405–414.

60. Jian L, Xie LP, Lee AH, et al. Protective effect of green tea against prostate cancer: a case-control study in southeast China. *Int J Cancer.* 2004;1:130–135.

61. University of Texas M.D. Anderson Cancer Center. Natural Standard. Natural Standard Database. Available at: http://www.naturalstandard.com/. Accessed May 8, 2004.

62. Cerhan JR, Putnam SD, Bianchi GD, et al. Tea consumption and risk of cancer of the colon and rectum. *Nutr Cancer.* 2001;41:33–40.

63. Sovak M, Seligson AL, Konas M, et al. Herbal composition PC-SPES for manage-
    ment of prostate cancer: identification of active principles. *J Natl Cancer Inst*
    2002;94:1275–1281.
64. Di Paola RS, Zhang H, Lambert GH, et al. Clinical and biologic activity of an estro-
    genic herbal combination (PC-SPES) in prostate cancer. *N Engl J Med.*
    1998;339:785–791.
65. Oh WK, George DJ, Hackman K, et al. Activity of the herbal combination, PC-SPES,
    in the treatment of patients with androgen-independent prostate cancer. *Urology.*
    2001;57:122–126.
66. Small EJ, Frohlich MW, Bok R, et al. Prospective trial, of the herbal supplement
    PC-SPES in patients with progressive prostate cancer. *J Clin Oncol.* 2000;18:
    3595–3603.
67. Pfeifer BI, Pirani JF, Hanmann SR, et al. PC-SPES, a dietary supplement for the treat-
    ment of hormone refractory prostate cancer. *BJU Int.* 2000;85:481–485.
68. Moyad MA, Pienta KJ, Montie JE. Use of PC-SPES, a commercially available supple-
    ment for prostate cancer, in a patient with hormone naive disease. *Urology.*
    1999;54:323–324.
69. Weiger WA, Smith M, Boon H, et al. Advising patients who seek complementary and
    alternative medical therapies for cancer. *Ann Int Med.* 2002;137:889–905.
70. Small EJ, Kantoff P, Nguyen S, et al. A prospective multicenter randomized trial of
    the herbal supplement, PC-SPES, vs. diethylstilbestrol (DES) in patients with ad-
    vanced, androgen independent prostate cancer (AiPCa) [abstract]. *Proc ASCO.*
    2002;May 18–21.
71. Heinonen OP, Albanes D, Virtamo J, et al. Prostate cancer and supplementation with
    alpha, tocopherol and beta carotene: incidence and mortality in a controlled trial.
    J Natl Cancer Inst. 1998;90:440–446.
72. Lamson DW, Brignall MS. Antioxidants in cancer therapy; their actions and interac-
    tions with oncologic therapies. *Alternative Medicine Review.* 1999;4:304–329.
73. Labriola DL. Possible interactions between dietary antioxidants and chemotherapy.
    Oncology (Huntingt). 1999;13:1003–1008,1011–1012.
74. PDR. *PDR for Nutritional Supplements.* Montvale, NJ: Medical Economics Company;
    2001.
75 Fletcher RH, Fairfield KM. Vitamin supplementation in disease prevention. Available
    at: http://www.uptodateonline.com/utd/content/topic.do?topicKey=genr_med/
    12211&type=A&selectedTitle=1~130 Accessed May 16, 2006.
76. Combs G. Status of selenium in prostate cancer prevention. *Br J Cancer.*
    2004;91:195–199.
77. Blackadar CB. Skeptics of oral administration of shark cartilage [letter]. *J Natl Can-
    cer Inst.* 1993;85:1961–1962.
78. Leitner SP, Rothkopf MM, Haverstick L, et al. Two phase II studies of oral shark car-
    tilage powder (SCP) in patients with either metastatic breast or prostate cancer re-
    fractory to standard treatment. *Proc ASCO.* 1998;18:A554.
79. Nagata C, Takatsuka N, Shimizu H, et al. Effect of soy milk consumption on serum
    estrogen and androgen concentrations in Japanese men. *Cancer Epidemiol Bio-
    markers Prev.* 2001;10:179–184.
80. Mousavi Y, Adlercreutz H. Genistein is an effective stimulator of sex hormone-
    binding globulin production in hepatocarcinoma human liver cancer cells and sup-
    presses proliferation of these cells in cluture. *Steroids.* 1993;58:301–304.

81. Habito RC, Montalto J, Leslie E, et al. Effects of replacing meat with soyabean in the diet on sex hormones concentrations in healthy adult males. *Br J Nutr.* 2000;84:557–563.

82. Wiseman H. Role of dietary phyto-oestrogens in the protection against cancer and heart disease. *Biochem Soc Trans.* 1996;24:795–800.

83. Williams JK, Clarkson TB. Dietary isoflavones inhibit in-vivo constrictor responses of coronary arteries to collagen-induced platelet activation. *Coronary Artery Dis.* 1998;9:759–764.

84. Akiyama T, Ishida J, Nakagawa S, et al. Genistein, a specific inhibitor of tyrosine-specific protein kinases. *J Biol Chem.* 1987;262:5592–5595.

85. Fotsis T, Pepper MS, Aktas E, et al. Flavonoids, dietary-derived inhibitors of cell proliferation and in vitro angiogenesis. *Cancer Res.* 1997;57:2916–2921.

86. Li D, Yee JA, Mcguire MH, et al. Soybean isoflavones reduce experimental metastasis in mice. *J Nutr.* 1999;129:1075–1078.

87. Yip I, Aronson W, Heber D. Nutritional approaches to the prevention of prostate cancer progression. *Adv Exp Med Biol.* 1996;399:173–181.

88. Meyer F, Bairati I, Shadmamni R, et al. Dietary fat and prostate cancer survival. *Cancer Causes Control.* 1998;10:1271–1275.

89. Bairati I, Meyer F, Fradet Y, et al. Dietary fate and advanced prostate cancer. *J Urol.* 1998;159:1271–1275.

INTERNET RESOURCES

SITE NAME: American Cancer Society
WEB SITE ADDRESS: www.cancer.org
MATERIAL AVAILABLE:
- Cancer research
- Treatment option
- Coping
- Cancer treatments
- Clinical trials

SITE NAME: American Foundation for Urologic Disease
WEB SITE ADDRESS: www.afud.org
MATERIAL AVAILABLE:
- Complete information on prostate cancer with description
- Glossary of medical terminology
- Examination, testing, and treatment information provided
- Quiz is available at end of formal presentation

SITE NAME: Association of Community Cancer Centers
WEB SITE ADDRESS: www.accc-cancer.org
MATERIAL AVAILABLE:
- Information on cancer centers
- Basic insurance information
- Treatments and standards

SITE NAME: Cancer-Links Prostate
WEB SITE ADDRESS: www.cancernews.com/
MATERIAL AVAILABLE:
- News reports on prostate cancer
- Links to other home and information pages
- Literature search—link to National Library
- Books on prostate cancer
- Listing of prostate cancer Web resources
- Clinical trial search—link to NCI of Medicine

SITE NAME: CancerNet information
WEB SITE ADDRESS: cancerweb.nci.ac.uk/cancernet.html
MATERIAL AVAILABLE:
- Information from PDQ
- Access to information from NCI's Office of Cancer Communication
- CANCERNET news and publications

SITE NAME: Center Watch
WEB SITE ADDRESS: www.centerwatch.com
MATERIAL AVAILABLE:
- Clinical trials listing service
- Listing of recently approved drugs
- Patient bookstore
- About research
- Drug directions
- Resources

SITE NAME: Web MD
WEB SITE ADDRESS: www.webmd.com
MATERIAL AVAILABLE:
- Articles on prostate cancer prevention, symptoms, and treatment
- Online support group
- Link to the Cleveland Clinic Web site—Your Guide to Prostate Cancer—
  www.clevelandclinic.org
- Link to information on clinical trials

SITE NAME: National Cancer Institute
WEB SITE ADDRESS: www.cancer.gov
MATERIAL AVAILABLE:
- NCI database
- Clinical trials data
- CancerNet
- Patient information
- Cancer information service

SITE NAME: National Prostate Cancer Coalition
WEB SITE ADDRESS: www.pcacoaliton.org
GOAL: Awareness outreach advocacy
MATERIAL AVAILABLE:
- Education
- Treatment info
- Advocacy
- Programs
- Newsletter (*Aware*)

SITE NAME: National Comprehensive Cancer Network
WEB SITE ADDRESS: www.nccn.org
MATERIAL AVAILABLE:
- NCCN prostate cancer treatment guidelines for patients
- Clinical trail links
- Cancer links

SITE NAME: OncoLink
WEB SITE ADDRESS: oncolink.upenn.edu
MATERIAL AVAILABLE:
- General information about cancer
- Questions and answers about
  prostate cancer
- Risk factors, prevention, and genetics
- Treatment options viewed
- Newspaper items pertaining to prostate cancer
  and related topics available for viewing or reprinting
- Can focus on prostate cancer
- Recommendations for screening
- Information on support groups

SITE NAME: ONS Online
WEB SITE ADDRESS: www.ons.org
MATERIAL AVAILABLE:
- Access to journal articles, discussion
  forums, excerpts from new books, and
  materials on genetics
- Patient education material
- Listing of ONS members
- Information regarding prevention and
  detection

continues

SITE NAME: Prostate info.com, AstraZeneca site
WEB SITE ADDRESS: prostateinfo.com
MATERIAL AVAILABLE:

- Disease
- Diagnosis
- Tests
- Clinical trials
- Treatment
- Risk factors
- Support
- Glossary

SITE NAME: Health Talk—Living with Hope
WEB SITE ADDRESS: www.htinet.com
MATERIAL AVAILABLE:

- Diagnosis
- Management
- Links to medical groups/advocacy, government agencies, education companies
- Treatment
- Research

SITE NAME: University of Michigan Comprehensive Cancer Center
WEB SITE ADDRESS: www.cancer.med.umich.edu
MATERIAL AVAILABLE:

- General information
- Staging information
- Resources
- Information regarding University of Michigan Comprehensive Cancer Center
- Clinical trials information
- Treatment options
- Links to NCCN

SITE NAME: National Prostate Cancer Coalition
WEB SITE ADDRESS: www.pcacoalition.org
MATERIAL AVAILABLE:

- Education
- Treatment info
- Advocacy
- Programs
- Newsletter—*Aware*
- Goals: awareness, outreach, advocacy

SITE NAME: The Prostate Forum
WEB SITE ADDRESS: www.prostateforum.com
MATERIAL AVAILABLE:

- Newsletter for patients-families written by Charles E. Myers, MD
- Side effects
- References
- Treatment issues
- Mechanisms of action
- Research
- Advocacy

SITE NAME: US TOO International, Inc. Prostate Cancer Education and Support
WEB SITE ADDRESS: www.ustoo.com
MATERIAL AVAILABLE:

- Information regarding organization
- Publications (updated monthly)
- Information on clinical trials
- Information can be requested
- Support groups
- Current treatment options
- Links provided to related sites

SITE NAME: The Prostate Net
WEB SITE ADDRESS: www.prostate-online.org
MATERIAL AVAILABLE:
- Education
- Advocacy/support
- Treatment
- Links

SITE NAME: The Association for the Cure of Cancer of the Prostate
WEB SITE ADDRESS: www.capcure.org
MATERIAL AVAILABLE:
- Overview
- Screening
- News
- Resources
- Detection
- Treatment
- Nutrition
- Personal stories

SITE NAME: Cancer Consultants
WEB SITE ADDRESS: www.cancerconsultants.com
MATERIAL AVAILABLE:
- Overview
- Screening
- Resources
- Prevention/early detection
- Treatment
- Clinical trials

Notes: NCI, National Cancer Institute; AFUD, American Foundation for Urologic Disease.

Source: Blecher C. Prostate cancer resources for patients, families, and professionals. In: Held-Warmkessel J., ed. *Contemporary Issues in Prostate Cancer: A Nursing Perspective.* 2nd ed. Sudbury, MA: Jones and Bartlett Publishers; 2006:416–440. Reprinted with permission from Jones and Bartlett Publishers.

index

Page numbers followed by t or f denote tables or figures respectively